D0710382

# The Natural History of Mania, Depression, and Schizophrenia

# The Natural History of Mania, Depression, and Schizophrenia

**George Winokur, M.D.**

The Paul W. Penningroth Professor of Psychiatry

University of Iowa College of Medicine

Iowa City, Iowa

**Ming T. Tsuang, M.D., Ph.D.**

The Stanley Cobb Professor of Psychiatry

Harvard Medical School

Boston, Massachusetts

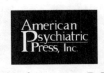

American Psychiatric Press, Inc.

Washington, DC
London, England

**Note:** The authors have worked to ensure that all information in this book concerning drug dosages, schedules, and routes of administration is accurate as of the time of publication and consistent with standards set by the U.S. Food and Drug Administration and the general medical community. As medical research and practice advance, however, therapeutic standards may change. For this reason and because human and mechanical errors sometimes occur, we recommend that readers follow the advice of a physician who is directly involved in their care or the care of a member of their family.

Copyright © 1996 American Psychiatric Press, Inc.
ALL RIGHTS RESERVED
Manufactured in the United States of America on acid-free paper
99  98  97  96    4  3  2  1
First Edition

American Psychiatric Press, Inc.
1400 K Street, N.W., Washington, DC   20005

**Library of Congress Cataloging-in-Publication Data**
Winokur, George.
    The natural history of mania, depression, and schizophrenia / by George Winokur and Ming T. Tsuang. — 1st ed.
        p.   cm.
    Includes bibliographical references and index.
    ISBN 0-88048-726-7
    1. Manic-depressive psychoses—Iowa—Longitudinal studies.
2. Schizophrenia—Iowa—Longitudinal studies.   3. Depression, Mental—Iowa—Longitudinal studies.   I. Tsuang, Ming T., 1931–
II. Title.
    [DNLM:   1. Psychotic Disorders—genetics.   2. Depressive Disorder—genetics   3. Schizophrenia—genetics.   WM 202 W776n 1996]
RC454.4.W56   1996
616.89'5—dc20
DNLM/DLC
for Library of Congress                                      95-21301
                                                                  CIP

**British Library Cataloguing in Publication Data**
A CIP record is available from the British Library.

# Contents

# Preface

In *Citizens*, a chronicle of the French Revolution, Simon Schama makes the point that the presentation of history varies in focus from themes to historical narrative. He presented the French Revolution as a narrative because he thought that showing the chronology made the circumstances more intelligible. In this account of the Iowa 500, we have presented the study as a narrative because we thought that this form would best serve the complicated subject matter. The organization of the book is unusual and does not revolve around traditional medical themes (i.e., clinical picture, outcome, familial illness). Rather it is organized around the temporal sequence of the separate studies that rose out of our central goals. Thus, this book begins with the conception of the Iowa 500, goes through the early subject selection and record analyses, reviews the field work with families and follow-up, and ends with a series of conclusions that fuse into a classification. Because of the specific qualities of the research, its systematic nature, its long-term follow-up, and evaluation of familial illness by both family history and family study methodology, we believe that the Iowa 500 has something significant to say about the affective disorders and affective psychoses as well as the chronic nonaffective psychoses. The study was done at a time when special new study designs and methods in the field, such as the separation of bipolar from unipolar illness, the advent of systematic criteria, and the use of blindness in assessment, became important aspects of research into the clinical aspects of psychiatry. There have been subsequent studies of the same issues, and, certainly, there had been previous studies dealing with some of the same problems. The findings from these studies will be compared, discussed, and questioned.

Where does the Iowa 500 fit in the nature of things psychiatric? In the early 1920s, two books by Professor Emil Kraepelin of Munich appeared in English. The first book was on dementia praecox, and paraphrenia, and the second book was on manic depressive insanity and paranoia. They were translated by R. Mary Barclay from the eighth German edition of Kraepelin's *Textbook of Psychiatry*. They were edited by George Robertson, M.D., F.R.C.P.(Edin.) who was the professor of psychiatry at the University of Edinburgh and physician to the Royal Asylum, Morningside. Both of these books were mainly descriptive, though they did contain some rudimentary statistics in terms of percentages. As Professor Kraepelin had essentially defined the major psychoses in these works, they were extremely influential. The study that we call the Iowa 500 deals with the same illnesses with particular emphasis on dementia praecox (schizophrenia) and manic depressive disease. Unlike Kraepelin's original books, it deals less with descriptive material and more with a systematic evaluation of the symptom picture, the course and outcome, and the family background. In a sense then, it is the second step that follows Kraepelin's epoch, separating the episodic and the deteriorating major psychoses. It has some advantage over recent studies in that the patients in the Iowa 500 were not given effective medications. Thus, the natural history is less influenced by treatment.

We present it as a book that should be interesting to everybody who deals with major psychiatric illnesses. This includes medical students, residents, psychiatrists, social workers, psychologists, and even ministers, who often have to deal with families that are concerned about such patients. It provides a baseline of what the professional might expect should treatment not be instituted. It also provides a clear indication of how the diagnoses of major psychiatric disorders might be made.

# Chapter 1

# Introduction to the Iowa 500 Study

Some inconstancy is inherent in psychiatric research and diagnosis; findings frequently point in opposite directions, creating a morass of contradictions and inconsistencies that leads to an attempt to reconcile the differences. Often, reconciliation is possible only by the observer who begins with unshakable conviction about the truth of one of the findings. Problems arise with the reliability of diagnoses made by two perfectly competent workers. At times, we face the question of what to do with patients whose characteristics and diagnoses change over time. We know that, in general, psychiatric illnesses breed true in families but that this is not invariable. We know that a family history of psychiatric illness can be useful but that a family study may be more precise. Having met reasonable criteria for an illness may not prove that the individual has the illness, but alternatively it is possible that if an individual has the illness and does not meet the criteria, precision in diagnosis may not be possible. The Iowa 500 study was conceived to deal with these problems.

1

In the early part of 1971, one of us (G.W.) visited the then University of Iowa Psychopathic Hospital before becoming head of the department of psychiatry. The weather was cold, and there were crusts of ice on the streets left over from late November of the year before. Like geological strata in an excavation, new generations of ice were layered on top of the oldest.

In the basement of the Psychopathic Hospital there was a record room that contained a gold mine of information. From the time that the hospital had opened in 1920, each patient's record had been kept in pristine condition. They were filed according to the date of first admission so that thousands of charts were easily available. At that time, we were beginning to think about a possible design for systematic studies in psychiatry, and we were intrigued by the opportunity of using these charts for an historical prospective study (currently referred to as "retrospective cohort" study) that encompassed both a 30- to 40-year follow-up and a systematic evaluation of familial illness.

The charts of these patients admitted in the 1920s, 1930s, and early 1940s were unusual. They were typewritten accounts of all psychiatric and social service interviews, progress notes, laboratory studies, discharge summaries, and, often, psychological test results. Also included were follow-up notes, which, for some patients, covered periods up to 20 years after discharge. Particularly unusual was the fact that there were verbatim transcripts of interviews with the head of the department of psychiatry at the University of Iowa for almost all of the patients. These transcripts contained of a variety of questions by the department head or other professors with answers by the patient. Often, these were three to five single-spaced pages in length; thus, the actual words of patients admitted 30–35 years before were preserved in these charts. The quality of material in terms of documenting symptomatology was quite sufficient for making diagnoses according to modern diagnostic criteria that had been published for research purposes.

Many of these charts were written by psychiatrists who became distinguished in the field of psychiatry (such as Andrew

Woods, Eric Lindeman, William Malamud, Jacques Gottlieb, Paul Huston, and Adolph Sahs). We reviewed hospital charts that were signed by researchers such as Fritz Redlich and Karl Rickels, who worked at the state hospitals in Iowa (Independence and Cherokee).

To understand the circumstances of the study, it is important to know something about the state of Iowa as the catchment area and the Iowa Psychopathic Hospital. The hospital was founded in 1920, around the same time that the Boston Psychopathic and Michigan Psychopathic Hospitals were built. The Iowa Psychopathic Hospital was funded by the state and was located on the University of Iowa campus. The staff of the hospital was designated as the department of psychiatry in the College of Medicine. For 70 years, this hospital has functioned continuously. There is a strong feeling of tradition in Iowa although it achieved statehood relatively late (1846). In the 1970s, we decided to change the name of the hospital from the Iowa Psychopathic to the Iowa Psychiatric Hospital. This had to be approved by the legislature in Iowa, and, for unknown reasons, about six members voted against the change in name, even though the term "psychopathic" was considered negative. Notably, the state hospitals had long before changed over to the more euphonious term of "mental health institutes."

The patients selected for the Iowa 500 had been admitted over a 10-year span from 1934 to 1944. It was relatively easy to reach our goal of 100 bipolar and 225 unipolar subjects between 1935 and 1940, but we had to go forward as far as 1944 to collect a consecutive admission group of 200 schizophrenics. The criteria for schizophrenia were extremely restrictive and picked up only the most severely ill patients. The patients with affective disorders (bipolar and unipolar) were also severely ill, but the criteria were less restrictive. Patients were referred from all locations of the state, but, because of transportation problems that existed at that time, only the patients most in need of care applied for admission. In this sense, Iowa Psychiatric was the primary admitting hospital for the state and was used for determining diagnoses and whatever acute treatment might be available. However, failure to recover usually necessitated transfer to one of the four chronic treatment state hospitals in Iowa. As an example of the severity of the cases, 64% of the bipolar probands (index cases) showed psychotic symptoms (i.e., delusions and hallucinations). Fifty-six percent of the unipolar patients (patients with depressions only) also showed such symptoms. In contrast, during the 1970s in the same hospital, 52% of bipolar patients and only 18% of unipolar depressive patients showed psychotic symptoms.

The people of the state take pride in that Iowa has always been a place where literacy has been emphasized. In the Iowa 500 groups, the premium placed on education may be noted from the high number of people who graduated from high school. It is a state with no huge pockets of poverty, although there have been times when the economy has been unstable. Iowa citizens have great respect for the work done at the university hospital, and, because of this, they tend to be accepting of interviews and helpful in providing material for follow-up studies. The lack of large pockets of dispossessed and discriminated people is a point in favor of cooperation by the subjects in a clinical study.

A number of aspects of the Iowa 500 study were unique. First, we started with a systematic evaluation according to prestated diagnostic criteria. In this case, "systematic" meant that we were attempting to be methodical in our work. All charts were subjected to the same questions, and all subjects were rediagnosed according to specific research diagnostic criteria. In addition, we decided to consider the possibility of a change of diagnosis and, therefore, needed a follow-up of the patients.

There are two reasons to do a follow-up study. The first reason is to determine the actual course of the specific illness. In this case, one would be interested in whether the illnesses were episodic with total remissions, episodic with incomplete remissions, chronic and stable, or chronic with a downhill, deteriorating course. Having made a criterion-based diagnosis, we were interested in what the course might be, but we were equally interested in the possibility that, over the course of many years, some of the patients might change diagnoses. Thus, a person might go from mania to schizophrenia, from depression to bipolar, or from depression to schizophrenia. Also, since the method used for this research was one of the first attempts at determining diagnoses by operational criteria, it was fundamental to validate these by conducting a long-term follow-up and family study.

In addition to those methodological improvements, all assessments were blind to the original diagnosis. Thus, the family history was assessed by an individual who did not know the diagnosis of the proband. This was also true for the family study where examiners went out into the community and interviewed both former patients and family members without knowing what the original research diagnosis might have been. Not knowing the diagnosis meant that the assessment of the outcome was blind and presumably not subject to preconceptions. This was made possible, in part, because of the selection of a control group, which will be discussed later.

One of the goals of the study was to determine the familial (possibly genetic) background of three illnesses: schizophrenia, bipolar illness, and unipolar depression. Thus, we found that it was necessary and useful to define major psychiatric illness at the outset, and we were not originally interested in patients who presented themselves as difficult cases to diagnose. We were able to compare such things as a family history to the family study methodology, but, inherent in the study, was also a possibility to do more exotic kinds of comparisons. Some aspects of the study to this day have not been investigated fully. For example, most of the probands were brought up by well parents, whereas all of the ill children of the probands were brought up by at least one ill parent. Thus, we could study the influence of being brought up by an ill parent on the development of an illness or even the frequency with which an illness occurs. Although the data are sufficient to answer these questions, up to this point we have not explored the differences that might be related to having been reared by an ill versus a well parent.

As we formulated a study where we would be able to determine stability of diagnosis over a period of 40 years, implicit in our thinking was the idea that the course of illness was as useful in making a diagnosis as the clinical phenomenology, perhaps even more so. This is another example of something that has not to this date been fully explored; which provides the greater resolving power, the clinical symptoms or the course of illness?

We had information from a systematic family history that was obtained by the social worker and often spanned four or five pages. As the patients were admitted between 1934 and 1944 and the study started in the early to mid-1970s, there was a plan to retrospectively follow-up the patients over 40 years. We were interested in being able to do both a family history and a family study, and we thought there would be enough stability of population in Iowa to make this feasible.

Why were the charts so good? The answer is simple—what else did the psychiatrist have to do? At that time, they spent most of their time observing and writing down their observations. In the period that the Iowa 500 patients were admitted, there was little in the way of treatment. Psychiatry was mainly a descriptive science, and good care necessitated both a very good evaluation and humanistic management. Some psychotherapy was done and some sedative drugs were used, but treatment was not comparable with what we can offer today. Much time, therefore, was devoted to documenting all clinical information in the charts.

It was this lack of effective treatment that provided us with the opportunity to evaluate the natural history of these major psychiatric illnesses. Treatment does not necessarily alter the symptoms or course of the illness because treatment that does not provide a desired effect can hardly change the clinical picture or outcome. In today's psychiatric climate, it would be next to impossible to study the natural history of bipolar or unipolar affective disorder or schizophrenia, but the methodology of the Iowa 500 allowed us to do just this.

The early researchers of the Iowa 500 study were people like Jim Morrison, who selected the patients and supervised the systematic recording of data. Although he did much of the work himself, he was aided by Raymond Crowe and John Clancy, who evaluated the records in a systematic fashion. Morrison could not count, so instead of selecting 500 patients, we amassed 525. We had originally planned to have 200 patients with schizophrenia, 200 patients with unipolar depression, and 100 patients with bipolar illness. As it happened, Morrison collected 225 unipolar patients. This turned out to be extremely useful in that some of the unipolar patients ultimately became bipolar, thereby reducing the number of unipolar patients to 203 and increasing the number of bipolar patients to 122. We had interesting experiences in the beginning. Barbara Norton, a social worker, carried out a pilot study to see how well we could follow-up the patients. For example, she would call a telephone operator in What Cheer, Iowa, and ask what had happened to Mrs. John Jones. The operator would say that she recalled Mrs. Jones but that she had left 12 years ago to go to Omaha where her husband worked in the meat packing industry. This kind of circumstance was common in the follow-up of the Iowa 500.

Of the first 50 patients who were followed-up by Mrs. Norton, 49 had obtainable information up to the present or to the time of death. Of the 50th patient, she only obtained information up to 15 years after the index hospitalization. Based on this experience, it looked as if a follow-up study was feasible. At one point, she came to us and said that one of the schizophrenic patients had committed suicide. We pointed out to her that schizophrenic patients never committed suicide. No doubt the patient had been misdiagnosed. When we asked her who made the diagnosis, she said that we had; we, therefore, had to consider the possibility that maybe we were wrong about schizophrenics never committing suicide. Never let it be said that we were too open-minded.

We recorded information from the charts and from the chart follow-up. Within a short time, Ming Tsuang came to the University of Iowa and became the director of the project. He functioned as head of the fieldwork and obtained funding for the long-term follow-up and family study. In fact, Tsuang was like a field marshal. He had a large map of the United States and a large map of Iowa, both with multicolored pins stuck in place for each of the patient and family interviews. It was an impressive sight. So, between 1971 and 1972, we started the Iowa 500 study. We were convinced that by making original research diagnoses according to systematic criteria and doing the long-term follow-up, this would result in reliable diagnoses that would enable us to perform a reliable family and genetic study. We knew that over a long period of time, a certain number of patients would become diagnostically less clear, rather than more clear, and so we had a category that was termed "undiagnosed." In the follow-up, we planned to evaluate chronic versus remitting course of illness, as well as whether the clinical presentation of the patients changed over time, necessitating a change in diagnosis. In addition, another goal was to look at the clinical variability of rigorously diagnosed psychiatric disease.

Over the years, we opened the data set to other researchers, which meant that the material was used to consider a variety of questions, many of which were not considered in the original plan. As an example, Bill Coryell used the data to examine the long-term course of patients with affective disorder who had psychotic symptoms and, then, compared these patients with those who had the same diagnosis but no evidence of psychosis. Thus, the authorship of the publications that resulted from the Iowa 500 study included not only the original researchers but also several other people who used the data for specific analyses. Because of this open policy, the usefulness and productivity of the study were greatly increased.

We called the study "The Iowa 500." We wanted a name that was memorable. The Iowa 500 opened its doors for business in mid-1971, 27–30 years after the patients in the study were admitted. The details of the study design, follow-up procedures, and results will be presented in the following chapters.

# Chapter 2

# Historical Perspective

The Iowa 500 study involved a system-atic evaluation of symptomatology and family history at time of admission to the hospital, a long-term follow-up of the patients, a family study that included personal examination, and the inclusion of a control sample that gave an estimate of psychiatric disorders in the population and served as a comparison group. It is the only study based on exception-ally complete records from the past with a follow-up in the pres-ent. A more common approach is that of a cross-sectional study design, which gathers information at one point in time. For a study such as the Iowa 500 to be acceptable, the original rec-ords must be carefully selected, elaborate, and complete. This was the case for the original admission material that was used to start the Iowa 500.

Other distinguished longitudinal and epidemiologic studies have been accomplished in psychiatry; however, none are ex-actly alike. This study specifically concerned diagnosis and clas-sification using the clinical picture, the family background, and the follow-up material as elements in a differential diagnosis. Other studies had differing goals but clearly deserve specific citation. Faris and Dunham (1939) evaluated mental disorders

9

in occupants of urban areas and concluded that the majority of schizophrenic patients, as well as patients with alcoholic psychosis or neurosyphilis, came from the inner city. This finding contrasted with that of manic depressive patients who were randomly distributed throughout the city.

The Sterling County study assessed psychiatric illnesses in a rural county in Nova Scotia during 1950. One of the important hypotheses noted was that the mental health of the community was dependent on the degree of integration or disintegration, the latter associated with psychiatric disorder. The investigators developed a structured interview and diagnosed patients based on the then-current criteria for psychiatric illness of the time (Leighton et al. 1959, 1963).

One of the best known studies of psychiatric illness was the Midtown Manhattan study in New York City (Srole 1975). Researchers evaluated several blocks and a sample of dwellings in midtown Manhattan. Each subject was interviewed in his or her home, and the material was rated by two psychiatrists for symptom formation and interference with social functioning. Twenty years later, a follow-up study was performed. Symptoms of psychiatric disorder and interference with social functioning were found in approximately 23% of the respondents. Hollingshead and Redlich (1958) studied psychiatrically ill patients who were treated in the New Haven, Connecticut, area. They found that social class status was inversely related to being a psychiatric patient and that types of mental illness varied with class position.

Two other epidemiologic and follow-up studies are notable. First is the Lundby study in Sweden, in which Essen-Möller (1956) evaluated the prevalence of mental illness as well as personality variance in the entire population. In this study, which occurred during the summer of 1947, four psychiatrists interviewed almost the entire population of Lundby. They found that 0.7% of the total population had schizophrenia. This percentage rose to 0.9% when the individuals suspected of having schizophrenia were taken into account. Second, Hagnell (1966) followed up the Lundby patients 10 years after they were first interviewed, providing a significant measure of the incidence of mental illness—the number of new cases occurring in a period of time. Hagnell found that the expectancy risk for schizophrenia (to age 60) was 2.1% for men and 0.7% for women. The estimated cumulative risk for being admitted to a mental hospital at some time was 4.1% for men and 5.5% for women. He noted that this was similar to the risk for being admitted to a psychiatric service in London (5%).

Perhaps the study that is most similar to the Iowa 500 is the Clinic 500 study, which was conducted at Washington University, St. Louis, Missouri (Guze et al. 1983; Martin et al. 1985). Both studies primarily concerned diagnosis and classification. In the St. Louis study, 500 subjects were identified as a representative cross section of outpatients attending a psychiatric clinic. Subjects and their relatives were given a structured interview. The patients were admitted to the study between 1967 and 1969, and follow-up interviews were conducted between 1973 and 1979, resulting in a 6- to 12-year follow-up for individual patients. Numerous significant findings in this study included a strong increase in the risk for familial schizophrenia for patients who met strict diagnostic criteria. Also, strictly diagnosed schizophrenic patients experienced intercurrent (secondary) depressions, but this did not affect the findings of either schizophrenia or primary depression in the relatives. In addition, some diagnoses were associated with excess mortality in the follow-up such as alcoholism, antisocial personality, drug addiction, homosexuality, organic brain syndrome, and schizophrenia. But excess mortality was not observed in patients with primary affective disorder. This study is directly comparable with the Iowa 500 study, although the range of diagnoses is far greater and the follow-up is far shorter. Nevertheless, it is a study that combined rigorous initial diagnoses, a follow-up, and a family study, all as part of the total effort. All of the Washington University patients were originally seen in an outpatient clinic, whereas all of the Iowa 500 patients were severely ill inpatients with schizophrenia, mania, or depression. Also, the Iowa 500 study had a nonpsychiatrically ill control group.

The Iowa 500 project was a landmark study with the primary goal of collecting long-term follow-up and family data on schizophrenia, mania, and depression groups. To provide a reliable baseline for comparison and to achieve blindness, the study also included a stratified random sample of nonpsychiatric surgical patients. The major objectives of the investigation were to accomplish a 30- to 40-year follow-up of all probands and control subjects and to interview personally, but blindly, all living subjects and their first-degree relatives. For use in personal interviews, a single structured objective interview form that could identify psychiatric disorders in patients, relatives, and control subjects was developed.

The purpose of this chapter is to offer a historical perspective in the development of the design and methods needed to reach the goals mentioned previously. When this project was first proposed in the early 1970s, the problem of diagnosis of psychiatric disorders for research and clinical purposes was paramount. Researchers needed to categorize diagnoses based on information such as clinical features, course and outcome, family and genetic background, and considerations of possible etiologies. Some work toward this objective had already been done, although most of the major studies had been performed abroad. Studies, such as Lundquist's 20-year follow-up of manic and depressive patients (Lundquist 1945) and Langfeldt's study of the differentiation between schizophreniform and schizophrenic psychosis (Langfeldt 1956) formed some of the basis for our thinking about the Iowa 500 study. Although these investigators took patients with clinically defined syndromes and followed them over the course of many years, their methods did not include a presentation of a systematic clinical evaluation of the index admissions or a detailed report of a systematic family study. Excellent studies of affective disorder had been published by Angst (1966) in Zurich and Perris (1966) in Sweden; however, these had been somewhat impressionistic in their evaluation of the affected family members. These researchers, along with Winokur et al. (1969), presented family data that demonstrated genetic factors in affective disorders and divided affective disorders into two types: manic-depressive (bipolar) disorder and depressive (unipolar) disorder.

Important work had also been done on schizophrenia, especially by Lindelius (1970) in Sweden. He and his colleagues analyzed rates of recovery, marriage, fertility, mortality, and morbidity risks among the relatives of schizophrenia and other psychiatric patients. They concluded that the study did not permit any unequivocal answers to the "nature/nurture" problem of schizophrenia. A primary reason for such difficulties was that diagnostic systems for major psychoses had not been standardized at the time of these studies.

Most of the studies completed before the late 1960s had not been performed blindly, and, as a consequence, there was the possibility that a halo effect had influenced the evaluation of the family history because investigators knew of the diagnoses of the probands. It was imperative to design a study of affective disorders and schizophrenia that integrated systematic clinical features, a systematic evaluation of the course, and a blind family interview with control subjects and their family members. Research and clinical diagnostic criteria, which incorporated such factors as clinical features, course, familial aspects, age at onset, and sex ratios, were desperately needed to define valid and reliable diagnostic categories.

Based on these concerns, one set of operational systematic diagnostic criteria was published in 1972 (Feighner et al. 1972). These criteria were based on previously published research findings and clinical experience. Earlier efforts at diagnosis had essentially drawn only from clinical experience. By using available systematically collected data, these new criteria marked a trend in psychiatric diagnosis and also formed the foundation for the Iowa 500 study.

The Feighner criteria for 14 psychiatric illnesses were developed by a group of psychiatrists from the department of psychiatry, Washington University School of Medicine, St. Louis. The significance of the development of these criteria was that they provided a framework for making comparisons among studies by using the same system to define the disorders under study.

In other words, the use of formal diagnostic criteria by a number of groups, regardless of whether their interests were clinical, psychodynamic, pharmacologic, or neuropsychological, would help solve the problem of whether patients described by different groups are comparable.

Although these criteria were the most efficient available at that time, large-scale studies were needed to validate the various disorders, especially the major psychoses. Five elements were considered important for establishing diagnostic validity in psychiatric illness: clinical description, laboratory studies, delineation from other disorders, follow-up studies, and family studies. The development of these criteria led us into the Iowa 500 study in which the diagnostic system described previously was applied to the chart material of patients seen in the 1930s and early 1940s at the University of Iowa Psychiatric Hospital. We selected 525 patients (200 schizophrenic, 100 manic, and 225 depressive), believing that these groups were reasonably "pure" and suitable for a follow-up and family study. Also included as part of the follow-up were 160 nonpsychiatric control patients.

It is important to recognize the quality of the clinical material that went into the Iowa 500 study. Considerable efforts were made to identify representative groups of depressive, manic, and schizophrenic patients and to make sure that they met the Feighner criteria. As has been noted elsewhere, patients who did not meet these criteria were excluded from the study. Patients who were clearly unusual, or for whom other diagnoses might be entertained, were also excluded from the study. In the early 1970s, at study inception, little data existed that had been published on rapid-cycling bipolar subjects, the influence of seasonality on depression, or on atypical depressive subjects. Thus, we collected no data that were relevant to these issues. Bipolar II patients—those with a short period of mania—were also excluded from the study, as they did not meet the length of time necessary for mania to fit the Feighner criteria. Such subjects were not addressed in the study, and it is not possible to obtain information about them at the present time.

All of the patients were hospitalized; most were severely ill and would be considered endogenous or melancholic. Criteria now used for melancholia (i.e., loss of interest or pleasure in activities or lack of reactivity to usually pleasurable stimuli [anhedonia]) were not recorded. But we did record other symptoms such as diurnal variation, early morning awakening, retardation or agitation, anorexia and weight loss, significant personality disturbance before the episode, and recovery from the episodes. In later chapters, we present the early clinical symptoms in light of the final diagnosis. Symptoms that are typically associated with endogenous depressions or melancholic depressions are so frequent in the affected patients of the Iowa 500 that there is little room to deal with highly specific symptom risk factors for outcome. However, it is possible to reevaluate the data to determine if symptoms, symptom clusters, or family background might be related to the course or end state.

The use of comparison groups in psychiatric research was not typically incorporated into research designs at the time we proposed the Iowa 500 study. We had to make a strong argument, therefore, as to the importance of control subjects in our study. We proposed that a random sample of 160 nonpsychiatric subjects be selected from patients admitted to the university hospital during the same time period as the psychiatric patients. A surgical control group consisting of patients admitted for appendectomy or herniorrhaphy was selected. The control subjects in the study reflected the same Iowa population from which the psychiatrically ill probands came. We proposed to study the control subjects with the same methods and procedures as employed while studying the probands. Thus, maximum comparability of the data from the two groups would be achieved.

Because of the importance attached to the control group in the Iowa 500 study, careful thought had been given to the actual procedure for selecting the group. The relative merits of matched control versus random control subjects were vigorously discussed by the research team members. The final conclusion was that a stratified random sample would be more appropriate for the design of the study and the hypotheses that needed to be tested. We created a stratified sample for age, sex, and socioeconomic status. Socioeconomic status was measured by whether patients paid for treatment themselves (private) or the state paid for the treatment (public) (29% males, public status; 14% males, private status; 46% females, public status; and 13% females, private status). The control subjects were selected in these same proportions matched for age. Eighty hernia patients and 80 appendectomy patients were chosen.

This was one of the best decisions we made concerning the project. The statistical implications of having baseline measurements for comparison for both probands and relatives were significant. The utility of nonpsychiatric control subjects in psychiatric research seems obvious today, but in the early 1970s, we needed to convince funding agencies that having control subjects was invaluable for our study.

The next major task for our group at Iowa was to design a single structured interview form that could be used to personally interview both probands and their first-degree relatives. The content and organization of our interview form were determined primarily by the goals and requirements of our long-term follow-up and family study of schizophrenia, mania, and depression. We named this instrument the Iowa Structured Psychiatric Interview (ISPI) (Tsuang et al. 1980c). ISPI provided detailed information about important aspects of psychiatric, social, and family history. Detailed information was gathered about the frequency and duration of symptoms that characterize the major psychoses. The instrument was designed to be administered by well-trained nonmedical personnel to facilitate its use in large-scale field studies. In addition, the ISPI was designed so that it could be used without any implication that the informant or the informant's relatives have any type of psychiatric history or current psychiatric problems.

Many interview forms that were available at the time were evaluated, but for our purposes we found them to be inadequate. Some of these forms presumed that the interviewer had an adequate amount of sophisticated experience in psychiatric

diagnosis. Others presumed that the study subject being interviewed was a psychiatric inpatient with a positive history of psychiatric illness. In our proposed Iowa 500 study, most of the
subjects actually interviewed would be nonpsychiatric (control
subjects and first-degree relatives). In addition, we wanted to
obtain a wider range of information than any existing interview
form provided. To record the desired information on social features, family history, psychiatric symptoms, psychiatric history,
precipitating factors, course and outcome of disease, and other
epidemiologic factors, the existing interview forms would have
been cumbersome and time consuming to administer. With
these objectives in mind, we designed a single structured interview form that would meet all of our specific needs. The form
contained a concise list of nonambiguous and nontechnical
questions providing necessary demographic, social, and familial
data and covered the symptoms developed at Washington University for schizophrenia, mania, depression, alcohol or drug
abuse, and selected neuroses.

To design an interview form that met all of our objectives,
members of the research team became thoroughly familiar with
the structured interview format. As prototypes, we used the
structured interview forms employed successfully by the World
Health Organization's International Pilot Study of Schizophrenia (World Health Organization 1973), the Present State Examination (Wing et al. 1974), and the Psychiatric History and
Social Description Schedules (World Health Organization
1973). The first draft of the interview form was generally over-
inclusive to allow for the widest possible range of opinion in our
research group. After much revision, the draft of the instrument
was tested for interrater reliability. Each of five psychiatrists
chose one psychiatric inpatient and conducted a videotaped interview with the patient. Each taped interview was shown to the
other four psychiatrists for their rating. Based on this exercise,
questions that proved reliable were retained; those that proved
unreliable were rejected; and others were rephrased to increase
reliability. Over a 1-year period, potential questions were revised
or deleted, and the interrater reliability testing was repeated

several times. The final version of the ISPI obtained a maximum amount of relevant objective data in a minimum amount of time. The approximate interview time was 20 minutes for an informant who was psychiatrically normal and 45 minutes for an informant who was experiencing or had experienced a psychiatric illness.

One of the goals in developing the ISPI was to make it linguistically precise so that the individuals administrating it could simply ask the study subject the question as written and accurately record the responses. Collecting reliable data could, therefore, be met by using well-trained interviewers. The first step in the training program was to set criteria based on the demands of the structured interview situation and the needs of the research project. Our interviewers had to be at ease meeting strangers and had to establish professional rapport in the homes of the study subjects. Because of the structured format of the interview instrument, it was unnecessary to require the interviewers to have formal training in psychiatry. After their selection, the interviewers were trained intensively in the mechanical administration of the ISPI form. The training course objectives were to prepare interviewers to conduct the structured interview in a sensitive but systematic manner, to record accurately any relevant information elicited from the study subjects, and to follow all guidelines on the ethics of the research project and the confidentiality of all personal information. One week was devoted to training the interviewers to use the ISPI. At the end of the week the interviewers were competent in using the instrument and lacked only the practical experience gained by interviewing in the field. An interrater reliability study immediately following the week of training provided the real validation of the training program. By the end of the training, we were confident that the interviewers would provide us with the objective and accurate information needed for the Iowa 500 research project.

Another unique aspect of this project was the procedure used at the time to consolidate and computerize the information collected from the interviews (Woolson et al. 1980). Effective use of the data collected using the ISPI depended directly upon careful and well-designed data management procedures such as transference of data from the ISPI forms to computer files and checking for validity and consistency of the responses. The ISPI form provided data from over 400 separate variables. This information was computerized to facilitate data analysis. The data management and editing methods developed for this project resulted in accurate analyses files that were used for many years to come.

The major significance of this project was the potential for outlining homogeneous disorders or syndromes within the general rubric of affective disorders and schizophrenia. Obtaining clinical material, follow-up material, and family data, along with information on control subjects, made it possible to separate specific types of schizophrenia and affective disorder. The definition of homogeneous subtypes had enormous importance for further biological, psychological, and social studies. At the time this study was funded in the early 1970s, it was the only large follow-up and family study of major psychoses to be initiated in this country. In addition, it was one of the first family studies of both schizophrenia and affective disorder consisting mainly of children and siblings, rather than with parents and siblings, as had been the case with almost all the studies completed before.

In summary, much of the work associated with this project set the stage for research in psychiatric epidemiology for years to come. The use of operational research criteria to select subjects allowed for comparison with future research. The selection of nonpsychiatric control subjects made it possible for interviewers to be blind as to the psychiatric status of the research subjects. The control subjects also provided a baseline for comparison with the major psychosis groups. The use of control subjects set the standard for future epidemiologic research. The logistics needed to trace and follow-up subjects from anywhere in the country was an immense task, and we believe this was one of the first attempts at such a large-scale psychiatric survey performed in the United States. At one point, we had eight full-time employees tracing the probands and their relatives by telephone. Data management techniques needed to handle such a large amount of incoming data were new in psychiatry at that time. Large customized computer programs had to be written to read the data and perform validity and consistency checks. Data management programs that are available today did not exist when we computerized our information. Finally, the statistical methodology developed to analyze the large data sets was unique in psychiatric research. Multivariate statistical techniques were used to analyze mortality, survival, outcome, symptomatology, and familial data. Our group was the first in psychiatric research to use proportional hazards methodology to analyze variables affecting mortality and survival in schizophrenia and affective disorders (Tsuang et al. 1980e). Thus, the procedures used to consolidate and analyze the information collected in the interviews were advanced for the time and established the basis for much future psychiatric research (Woolson et al. 1980).

# Chapter 3

# Background Findings in Course and Follow-Up of the Affective Disorders and Schizophrenia

The natural history of an illness is its course when undisturbed by effective treatment. It should encompass precipitating and predisposing factors as well as epidemiology and outcome. In the case of psychiatric illnesses, the major problem revolves around the fact there is considerable heterogeneity. A similar syndrome may be seen in a variety of illnesses, and the same illness may have several guises. Until we have defined a homogeneous illness, it may not be possible to define the natural history with complete confidence, although a general assessment may be feasible. A problem of this kind occurs in the affective disorders. In 1966, bipolar affective (manic-depressive disease) disorder was separated from unipolar depressive (depressive disease) disorder. Prior to this time, the strong possibility of two diseases was considered but not taken seriously enough to separate the groups in studies of depression. With the separation of bipolar from unipolar affective disorder, however, certain characteristics of the two diseases became clear. Bipolar illness, in addition to showing both mania and depression (as opposed to the unipolar illness, which showed only depressions), was also likely to exhibit an earlier onset and more episodes or attacks (Winokur 1973a). Though not part of the course specifically, it was clear that bipolar patients showed both a higher degree of familial affective disorder and a higher number in the family affected with mania.

By the time that the separation of bipolar from unipolar illness had been accomplished, it had become almost impossible to do a natural history study because, at that point, effective treatment was available for both depressions and manias. Thus, in exchange for a more precise diagnosis and treatment that worked, the ability to do a natural history study became more difficult.

By contrast, treatment of schizophrenia is often helpful in management but may not change the course of the illness. Heterogeneity remains a major problem in schizophrenia, and diagnostic stability may vary over time. At one point, patients with delusional disorder—an illness that is characterized by implausible but not impossible types of delusions—might have been considered a part of schizophrenia. Newer data, however, suggest that patients with delusional disorder have a different family history as well as a different course of illness from that found in schizophrenia. Schizophrenic patients may do far less well in regard to productive living than patients with delusional disorder (Kendler et al. 1981; Opjordsmoen 1989; Winokur 1977). However, there may be even more important aspects of heterogeneity. Paranoid schizophrenics—patients with delusions and hallucinations but no formal thought disorder, no motor symptoms, and no marked affect change—may have a different course of illness than hebephrenic-catatonic schizophrenics who become ill earlier and who have a much greater chance of becoming incapacitated for independent life. (Kendler et al. 1984). Finally, based on DSM-III criteria (American Psychiatric

Association 1980), the lifetime prevalence rate for schizophrenia ranged from 1%–1.9% (L. Robins et al. 1984).

Nevertheless, even with the problems of heterogeneity and the influence of effective treatment, it is possible to make some general statements about the natural history of bipolar and unipolar illness and schizophrenia.

Coryell and Winokur (1992) reviewed course and follow-up studies of bipolar and unipolar affective disorder, and the points made about the course and outcome in affective disorder patients are reviewed in great depth in that review. These follow-up studies are of relatively recent vintage because the separation of bipolar and unipolar illness was not accomplished until Leonhard suggested it in 1962, and Angst in Zurich, Perris in Sweden, and Winokur and Clayton in St. Louis, all in 1966, presented family differences between the two entities, which supported the strong possibility that they were separate disorders (Angst 1966; Angst and Perris 1968; Perris 1966; Winokur and Clayton 1967). While reviewing data on bipolar illness, these researchers found that certain aspects about the course became clear. Generally, the mean age at onset for bipolar illness is around 30 and a substantial number of patients become ill during adolescence. There is some question as to whether the onset of bipolar illness may occur prior to puberty, though some studies have suggested that it does (Winokur et al. 1969). Bipolar illness may begin with a mania but may equally well begin with a depression. Both syndromes are followed by a very specific immediate course of illness. About 50% of bipolar patients begin with a reasonably short depression that lasts a couple of months and then becomes a mania. Another group starts with a mania and ends with a somewhat longer depression of about 9 months. Not only do bipolar patients show a biphasic course, but some show a triphasic course that starts with a depression and is succeeded by a mania, which in turn is followed by a long depression.

Manic episodes prior to the years of effective treatment lasted between 7 and 13 months, but for patients who were followed after 1945 (at which time there was clear evidence of effective treatment, e.g., electroconvulsive therapy [ECT]), episodes became much shorter and were usually terminated between 1.8 and 2.7 months. There had been patients, however, who were chronic and remained ill with mania for several years (Wertham 1928). Although these are still encountered by clinicians, they are infrequent; however, it is possible that older patients have longer episodes. At the extreme, Wertham (1928) reported that of 2,000 hospitalized manic patients, 14 (.7%) had symptoms that lasted longer than 5 years. Because this is such an old study, readers might be interested in how mania was defined. There were no systematic criteria in 1928, but the description of mania was already quite well known. Kraepelin (1904) published *Lectures on Clinical Psychiatry,* in which he described maniacal excitement; the patient quickly enters the room, his voice loud, and he answers immediately and soon takes over the conversation. He describes himself as "happy as a king." He talks a lot and with considerable animation and loses the thread, bringing in new, irrelevant details. His frame of mind is joyous, and he jokes a lot. Prior to coming into the hospital, he had gone to taverns and "disreputable houses" and behaved very extravagantly, but he did not consider himself ill. Kraepelin described an unstable train of thought, an exalted changing mood, motor unrest, and a passion for talk. The patient, in time, as his excitement mounted, developed senseless delusions. Diagnostic criteria, at the time, were essentially contained in White's "Outlines of Psychiatry" (Nervous and Mental Diseases monographs, New York, 1935). Mania manifested itself by three cardinal symptoms: flight of ideas, psychomotor excitement, and emotional excitement. Thus, although we've come a long way in diagnosis of mania, we might say "plus ça change, plus c'est la même chose." Other investigators presented data indicating that about 4%–11% of manic patients did not recover over a long follow-up and, thus, could be considered as having had a chronic course.

Early studies of manic (bipolar) patients over a long follow-up period suggested that about half had experienced only one attack (Lundquist 1945). One of the reasons for this substantial proportion may be that the early studies dealt primarily with subsequent hospitalizations. In more recent studies, the occurrence of the single episode course is unusual. Studies that were done after the 1960s suggest that 0%–26% of patients have a single episode course. In fact, Angst and co-workers (1973), in a fairly long follow-up of 1–12 years, found that only .5% of bipolar patients had a single episode. Some observations have led to the conclusion that episodes occur more closely together as time goes on. Also, some data suggest that episodes cluster over time and may ultimately "burnout" as the individual ages (Saran 1969; Winokur 1975b). The phenomenon of frequent shifts between mania and normality, or between mania and depression, is called rapid cycling. The usual definition of rapid cycling encompasses the idea that the individual has had four or more episodes in a year. The literature suggests that females are more likely to show rapid cycling than males (Coryell et al. 1992).

Bipolar illnesses manifests itself by multiple episodes. A high proportion of individuals may suffer from interepisode morbidity, being generally depressed over long periods of time. This kind of course could be called "episodic with intercurrent morbidity" or "partial remission with episodes." During the follow-up, however, a large number of patients are well between episodes. Thus, intercurrent morbidity is not an invariable finding in bipolar patients. In an assessment of long-term prognosis for bipolar illness, about 15%–45% were considered not socially recovered or not free of symptoms for any length of time and were considered "poor" according to overall functioning. Alternatively, 11%–78% were considered recovered, had an absence of psychiatric symptoms at follow-up, or were regarded as "good" in overall functioning. Stability of diagnosis in bipolar illness is relatively good with only about 8%–9% of patients with a subsequent diagnosis of schizophrenia (Lundquist 1945).

The ultimate outcome—death—was far more important in bipolar illness prior to the advent of effective treatment. About one-fifth of admitted manic patients died of cardiac problems or "exhaustion." In more modern times, natural causes are not related to any large excess mortality; but suicide is high among bipolar patients, although it has been reported that eventual suicide in bipolar patients is lower than in unipolar patients (Black et al. 1987a, 1987b).

Some patients with mania have subsequent attacks that are always manic and have been termed "unipolar" manic patients. It is quite likely that they should not be considered separately in that their family history is the same as patients who have both manias and depressions. Also, it is possible that some of the patients who are said to have unipolar mania have had depressions that were mild and not recognized. It should be noted that the largest group of patients with unipolar affective disorder are unipolar depressive, which differs from bipolar disorder in course of follow-up. In dealing with unipolar depression, it is necessary to recognize that some patients begin depressed and become bipolar. This switch from unipolarity to bipolarity probably occurs in 10% of the cases (Winokur and Wesner 1987). Estimates of the lifetime prevalence of major affective disorder in the general population range from 6.1%–9.5% (L. Robins et al. 1984).

Onset of unipolar depression, ordinarily in the late 30s or early 40s, is usually later than in bipolar illness. Onset in bipolar illness is very acute, with an individual going from wellness to hospitalization in a much shorter time than occurs in unipolar depression. Unipolar depression tends to have a more subacute type of onset, and symptoms may last for weeks or months before the community or the family notices that hospitalization is necessary. Unipolar depression varies in length, but in modern times the data suggest that 80% of unipolar patients recover from their depression within 40–50 weeks and 50% of unipolar depressive patients recover within 20 weeks (Coryell and Winokur 1992). On the other hand, 50% of bipolar patients recover from their mania within 10 weeks, and by 30 weeks 80%–100% have recovered from their mania. There is some possibility that a late age at onset in females is associated with a longer duration in unipolar depression (Winokur 1973b). The old concept of involutional melancholia included, as part of the definition, a late onset of a unipolar depression with a lot of nihilistic delusions and a long course when untreated. It was in that group of patients—the involutional melancholics—that ECT showed its greatest effect. Before ECT, patients with involutional melancholia stayed in the hospital for years; however, after the advent of ECT, patients were discharged much more rapidly and essentially in a recovered condition. Unipolar depressive patients recover in 83%–98% of the cases in a 5-year follow-up. Earlier studies with substantial follow-up suggest that 18%–61% of cases had a single episode course, but later follow-up studies suggest that, at 5%–55%, this is less common than was previously thought. Though the prognosis in unipolar depression is better than that in bipolar illness, long-term studies suggest that, over time, 14%–19% continue to have depressive symptoms that are incapacitating for employment in some degree. What seems clear about unipolar depression is that it is an episodic illness in which there are fewer episodes, and the severity is somewhat less than in bipolar illness. The change of diagnosis from unipolar depression to bipolar depression is substantial, about 10%, but the change from unipolar depression to schizophrenia is relatively small at 0%–6%. Mortality is high in unipolar depression, mainly because of the propensity for suicide, with risk highest during the first 1 or 2 years after hospitalization and becoming lower with time. There is a high degree of both unnatural and natural deaths in unipolar depression; the excess of natural deaths is usually the result of individuals entering the hospital with both medical and psychiatric illness (Black et al. 1987a). It is certainly possible that individuals with two diseases are more likely to be admitted to a hospital, and this factor may be the reason for an increased mortality rate from natural causes.

A recent development in studies of the natural history of treated unipolar patients has attempted to separate patients into those with neurotic depression versus those with endogenous depression and those with delusional depression versus those with nondelusional depression. It is also possible to separate unipolar depressive patients into those with a specific kind of family background (i.e., a family background of depression only, a family background of alcoholism with or without depression, and a family background with no psychiatric illness [sporadic]). Depressed patients with a family background of alcoholism (depression spectrum disease) are more likely to have an early onset and to experience significant social problems (Winokur 1982).

Patients who have an admixture of psychotic schizophrenic symptoms and affective symptoms are often called schizoaffective. Generally, such patients have a better outcome than patients with unequivocal schizophrenia. The concomitant presence of these two types of symptoms often makes diagnosis difficult, and a history of schizophrenia-like symptoms has been associated with a poorer outcome than that of patients with only affective symptoms. In general, an acute schizoaffective disorder follows a course like that of affective disorders, whereas a chronic onset of schizoaffective disorder has an outcome more like that of chronic schizophrenia (Tsuang and Dempsey 1979; Winokur 1989).

Follow-up studies in schizophrenia are subject to considerable controversy because the presence of psychotic symptoms may not a schizophrenic make. If the illness is acute in onset, the presence of schizophrenic symptoms does not necessarily lead to a schizophrenic course of illness. Acute onset schizophrenia may have far more in common with the affective disorders, both bipolar and unipolar, than with the chronic schizophrenias. It is quite possible that the presence or absence of affective or schizophrenic symptoms is less important than the mode of onset, acute versus chronic, or the course as defined by either full remission or chronicity. Some investigators (Stephens et al. 1960; Vaillant 1964) have attempted to separate patients with psychotic and schizophrenic symptoms into good and poor prognosis types. In these studies, good prognosis schizophrenia was typified by such factors as acute onset, the presence of affective symptoms, and a family background of affective disorder. Using such criteria, Stephens and co-workers reported that, of a group of schizophrenic patients, 18% of the poor prognosis patients had recovered in 5 years as compared with 80% of the good prognosis group. Vaillant found that in the short-term there was a 10% remission rate among the poor prognosis group (6–12 months). However, in his poor prognosis group, followed for 8–15 years, 16% suffered remission. Valliant's good prognosis group showed a rise in remission rate from 64% at 12 months to 84% in the long-term follow-up. These terms—good and poor prognosis schizophrenia—may constitute separate or autonomous illnesses.

The follow-up studies in schizophrenia are probably less affected by treatment than those in the affective disorders, the question being whether treatment changes the course of schizophrenia or is simply useful in managing the illness without really altering either the symptoms or the course very much (Chandler and Winokur 1989) is questionable. Certainly, there are data to suggest that once the illness is well established, treatment for schizophrenia does not produce remissions. In any event, because of diagnostic uncertainty, it is possible that some affective disorder patients are diagnosed as schizophrenic at some point and some schizophrenic patients are diagnosed with affective disorder on occasion. This would mean that a small proportion of chronic schizophrenic patients might remit, but the question of the remission would be influenced by the precision of the diagnosis. Of course, it remains possible that some patients with schizophrenia may recover from their illness.

The question of the quality of improvement in schizophrenia is a vital issue that could tell us something about the nature of the illness. There are a series of questions that need to be answered and that have not been specifically addressed in the current literature. One of the questions is whether it is possible for an individual to have a schizophrenic syndrome lasting several months to a year from which he or she recovers and shows no sign of disability or defect state. If this is possible, it suggests that schizophrenia is, in some cases, a remitting illness. The next question is whether an individual might have psychotic or schizophrenic symptoms consistently for a period of 5 years and, when followed up, be completely well with no evidence of a defect state or any symptoms. A course of this kind would suggest that not only is the illness remitting, but chronic long-term changes may be reversible. Several studies have dealt with the quality of improvement in schizophrenia. There is no doubt that, over time, some schizophrenic patients would partially improve so that their symptoms were less in evidence. But this does not necessarily mean that they are well, since they still may be suffering from a defect state that is stabilized and with which they have learned how to cope. Recent studies, however, have attempted to deal with the question of remission from schizophrenia.

Some studies examined the quality of life of a patient who has been followed up for a schizophrenic illness. Bleuler (1974), in a follow-up of 208 schizophrenic patients over the period of 1942–1964, noted that, on the average, schizophrenic patients do not get worse after 5 years and might show some tendency to improve. His major point was that such patients do not progress necessarily to severe dementia. He found that long-standing remission or recovery was unrelated to treatment. Most specifically, he noted that, after many years, some patients who had been incoherent began to speak in a normal fashion and other patients who were markedly apathetic started to interact in a social manner. However, it is impossible to determine whether patients who make this marked improvement are actually well or whether they might have some kind of mild or moderate defect state. Chiompi (1980) followed 289 patients for almost 37 years, and he found that the global outcome was favorable in 49% of the patients who had been followed at least 5 years. Twenty-seven percent were in remission and 22% had minor symptoms. The diagnosis was made according to Bleulerian criteria and did not include a poor outcome as being an obligatory criterion. Again, one could raise questions as to how well these patients were. With regard to diagnosis, precision is not good enough to have a 100% certainty; thus, there would be some disagreement on initial diagnosis. It would have been useful to have a description of the patients who were considered to be in remission and a comparison of their behavior with that of people matched for age and sex in the population. Probably the most optimistic study was published by Harding and co-workers (1987) who followed 118 patients over a period of 32 years who were admitted to the Vermont State Hospital in the United States. After rediagnosing these patients according to the criteria for schizophrenia in DSM-III, they found that one-half to two-thirds showed improvement or recovered and also noted that 68% of 82 subjects who met DSM-III criteria for schizophrenia at index admission did not display any further schizophrenic symptoms—negative or positive—at follow-up. Moreover, 45% had no psychiatric symptoms at all. Thus, one could ask whether other diagnoses besides schizophrenia might have been entertained in this group.

One of the more important studies was published by Johnstone and co-workers (1984) who followed, over a period of 5–9 years, 120 schizophrenic patients who met Feighner criteria for schizophrenia and were discharged from the hospital after having been hospitalized for schizophrenic symptoms. Eighteen percent had no significant symptoms and functioned satisfactorily, whereas 50% had a definite set of psychotic symptoms, and the remainder were somewhat in between. She reported two subjects that she considered well. One of these was a 28-year-old nightclub dancer who was living a perfectly productive life, and another subject was a 36-year-old single man who worked as a clerk and had some social interest, mainly in church. Each of these subjects was apparently hospitalized on one occasion, and it is possible that they are examples of patients who had schizophrenia, which arrested early and was associated with no obvious defect. All of the studies show a rather high degree of schizophrenic patients having chronic illness. However, these last studies suggest that the prognosis is not as grim as had been previously thought. The data collected from the Iowa 500 study enabled us to look again at some of the unipolar, bipolar, and schizophrenic patients who had been followed up and to determine what they look like compared with each other as well as what the quality of improvement or remission might be.

Like all studies, the Iowa 500 had some inherent biases such as the patients being severely ill in addition to being admitted to a university hospital. In the mid-1930s to mid-1940s, travel was not as easy as it is in the present, and only the most severely ill patients came to the hospital. This observation is supported by the disproportionate number of subjects with psychotic symptoms among the depressed and manic patients. The advantage of this selection bias is that there was little argument as to whether or not these patients meet systematic diagnoses. Essentially, the Iowa 500 study deals with patients who were untreated, and, consequently, the findings of the study immediately can be compared with the results of treatment studies of severely ill patients. To be considered effective, treatment of comparable patients must result in a better course and outcome than are found in this study.

# Chapter 4

# Family Background in the Major Functional Psychoses

For the affective disorders and schizophrenia, no proximal etiology is known. A proximal etiology would accurately describe the pathophysiology of the disease as well as the precipitating factors that caused the disease to become manifest. The distal etiology, however, is available, mainly familial and possibly genetic. An illness that has a genetic background shows the phenomenon of "breeding true," which means that, in an illness with a genetic etiology, ill members of the family will show what is easily diagnosed as the same illness present in the index case. Schizophrenia appears more frequently in the families of schizophrenic patients, and affective disorder patients show more affective disorders in their families than would be expected in the general population. Though the illnesses may not be exact copies of each other, they are usually similar in symptoms, course, premorbid characteristics, response to treatment, and, in some cases, laboratory findings. In addition to the clustering of illnesses in the same family, twin studies should reveal that monozygotic twins are more likely concordant than dizygotic twins because the monozygotic twins share 100% of their genes and the dizygotic twins share only 50%.

Often, in a genetic illness, disorders of the same functional system may be more prevalent in the families of the index cases. Generally, the functional system that is impaired in the affective disorders or schizophrenia is the central nervous system, and it is conceivable that other central nervous system or behavioral illnesses may be found more frequently in the families of affective disorder patients and schizophrenic patients than would be expected by chance in the general population. For example, alcoholism could conceivably be more frequent in the families of schizophrenic and affective disorder patients than in the families of normal control subjects. The family study component of the Iowa 500 project was designed to test for "breeding true" in schizophrenia and affective disorder.

Characteristics, like those described previously, suggest (but do not prove) a genetic factor in an illness. Whereas all genetic illnesses should show such findings, the findings may not be specific to a genetic illness. Etiologies such as infections or nutritional problems could lead to the same sorts of relationships that appear genetic. There are three ways one could prove a genetic factor. First, an adoption study (where children born of parents with an affective disorder or schizophrenia were separated early or at birth) could provide evidence of a genetic factor. Thus, adoptees having an increased frequency of the same illness as the biological parents would be clear evidence of a genetic factor. Similarly, if ill adoptees showed an increased frequency of the same illness in biological parents but no increased amount of the illness in adoptive parents, the data would support a genetic etiology. The second method of testing a genetic component is the twin study. Identical twins separated at birth, but still showing an increase of concordance over that expected in dizygotic twins, would also be a conclusive factor in proving a genetic background. Finally, if most of these illnesses manifested a demonstrable association or linkage to a known genetic marker, there would be no question about a genetic background.

A proven genetic background does not necessarily mean that other factors are not relevant to the illness. A multitude of environmental factors may influence the appearance of the illness or, in fact, may even prevent or make more likely the manifestation of the disease. It is not unusual that the major psychoses are multifactorial in origin, with both genetic and environmental factors playing significant roles. Relevant environmental factors may include exposure to toxins, medical illness, and dietary factors as well as psychosocial factors.

The advantages of genetic studies in the affective disorders or schizophrenia are clear. A positive finding suggests an unequivocal biological factor. This provides a starting place for further studies into the etiology and pathophysiology of the illness. In fact, if linkage with a known genetic factor were demonstrated, it may be possible in a stepwise fashion to approach a specific gene involved in transmission and describe the *modus operandi* of that particular gene. Of course, this has not yet been done in psychiatry, but it is reasonable to think that this kind of research might lead to major breakthroughs in understanding psychiatric illnesses.

There are two other reasons to be interested in genetic research in psychiatry. It is useful to know about a family background in terms of diagnosis of the family member. Thus, if one family member has an illness of schizophrenia and there is a problem with a difficult diagnosis of another family member, it is likely that this other ill family member may have the same disease. If an individual appears in the hospital with both schizophrenic and manic symptoms and has a clear family history of bipolar illness, it is conceivable that the patient's illness is an aberrant bipolar presentation. Coming from a family with one of these illnesses puts a person at high risk for the same illness; therefore, we could predict the onset of such an illness with increased certainty. If we had a good idea of how to prevent such psychiatric illnesses as the affective disorders or schizophrenia, we could bring into play preventive measures to ward off the illness.

For the clinical psychiatrist, however, there is a second reason to be interested in genetic studies since illnesses such as unipolar depression may be quite heterogeneous. For that matter, this could also be true of bipolar illness and schizophrenia, although unipolar illness is particularly likely to be an example of heterogeneity. After all, the diagnosis of unipolar depression is not the diagnosis of the disease but rather the diagnosis of a syndrome. This syndrome may be seen in a variety of diseases, and it may vary from one disease to another by a greater or lesser extent. By defining psychiatric illness according to the type of transmission or the type of familial background, we may be able to get closer to the concept of an autonomous disease. This would be extremely useful because there is reason to believe that treatment would differ depending on which specific disease was involved, although the clinical presentation may be similar.

In the last quarter of this century, there has been a renaissance of interest in genetic and family studies within psychiatry. To a large extent, this stems from the useful separation of bipolar and unipolar affective disorder mainly on the basis of familial differences, which stimulated further studies in both schizophrenia as well as the affective disorders themselves.

Numerous reviews have dealt with these issues, including a particularly useful evaluation of genetic studies in schizophrenia that was presented by Gottesman and co-workers (1987). These authors reviewed schizophrenia throughout the world and found the following proportion of family members who were affected with the same disease: children, 9.4%–12.8%; siblings, 7.3%–9.3%; monozygotic twins, 44%–46%; dizygotic twins, 12.1%–13.7%; half siblings, 2.9%–6.0%; nieces and nephews, 2.7%–3.5%; grandchildren, 2.8%–5%; and first cousins, 1.6%–2.4%.

As one goes from a sharing of 100% of genes to 50%–25%, there is a decrease in the proportion of ill relatives. Some investigators have attempted to divide schizophrenic patients with and without a family history into two groups that are separable from each other in certain ways. This poses a problem, however. If each relative has a certain risk of having the same illness, the more relatives one contacts, the more likely that a positive family history will be found. Thus, to separate schizophrenic patients into family history positive and family history negative groups, one would have to control for the number of family members that were investigated in both groups. This is not impossible, although independence within a family may present a problem. Thus, if an individual has one ill member of the family, it is very likely that he or she will have another ill member of the family, and the more ill members of the family that one finds, the more probable that the next person investigated will be ill. Monozygotic concordances are higher (52%) when a high number of negative symptoms are found than when a low number of negative symptoms are reported (36%). This suggests either a continuum of severity in schizophrenia or, alternatively, two types of schizophrenia: one that has a weak familial or genetic element and one that has a higher family history. Though we cannot say that the problem of family history positive and family history negative schizophrenia is a useful dichotomy, it is certainly worth continuing study.

Adoption studies lend support to the view that there is a genetic factor in schizophrenia. Kety and co-workers (1975) performed such a study in Denmark in which they found that families of adopted schizophrenic subjects had far more schizophrenia than did the families of adopted control subjects. Also, the biological families of the schizophrenic adoptees had far more schizophrenia than did the adoptive families. An assessment of identical twins, both separated and unseparated at birth, was published by Slater and Cowie (1971). Whether or not the twins were separated at birth, they had a similar expectancy of concordance for schizophrenia (63%). Thus, there seems to be an unequivocal genetic factor in schizophrenia, but the strength of this contribution is not as yet known.

In the affective disorders, there has also been a large amount of work studying families and twins. This was reviewed by Nurnberger and associates (1986), who evaluated a large number of studies that began with bipolar and unipolar probands. The lifetime prevalence of affective illness in first degree relatives of bipolar probands is 9%–41%. This is the proportion of illness in relatives when corrected for the age of risk for bipolar illness and the age of the relatives. These figures include both bipolar and unipolar relatives; most studies show that family members of bipolar probands are more likely to have unipolar depression (two-thirds of ill relatives) than bipolar illness (one-third of ill relatives). However, the rate of bipolar illness is considerably higher than one expects in a unipolar proband sample. Thus, the morbid risk for bipolar illness in the families of bipolar probands varies between 2.5%–17.7%, but in the family members of unipolar probands it varies between .3% and 4.1%. For all affective illness in the families of unipolar probands, lifetime prevalence varies between 6% and 20.1%. In studies of normal probands, lifetime prevalence for combined bipolar and unipolar affective illness in family members varies between .9% and 7.4%.

A number of comparisons of affective illness in monozygotic twin pairs and dizygotic twin pairs have been made. Concordance in the dizygotic twins varies between .0% and 23.6%. Concordance for monozygotic twin pairs varies between 33% and 92.6%. Summing up the studies, the concordance for monozygotic twins is 65% and 14.0% for dizygotic twins. Perhaps the best of all of the recent twin studies has been that of Bertelsen (1979). For affective disorders as a whole, he reported a concordance rate for monozygotic twins of 58.3% and 17.3% for dizygotic twins. The most interesting aspect of the Bertelsen study is that the concordance rate for bipolar monozygotic twins is higher than the concordance rate for unipolar monozygotic twins. This suggests that unipolar illness is a heterogeneous group or that it is "less genetic" than the bipolar group. If some unipolar patients were produced by nongenetic factors, this would account for the difference in concordance rate in monozygotic twins. Also, if there were some other type of illness (differential expressivity) that was related to unipolar depression genetically, that would also account for the difference in concordance rate in monozygotic twins. Interestingly, in a recent study of primary unipolar depressive patients compared with control subjects, females were more likely to have a family history of alcoholism than female controls (Winokur and Coryell 1991), suggesting that at least one type of depression is related to alcoholism, which is the way that the illness tends to express itself in males.

These findings indicate that there is a genetic factor in many cases of affective disorders. However, stronger evidence exists for the presence of a genetic factor in affective disorder. Price (1968) was able to cull from the literature 12 cases of monozygotic twins raised apart in which at least one twin had either bipolar or unipolar affective disorder. In that series, eight pairs (67%) showed concordance, which is quite similar to the findings in unseparated monozygotic twins. Schulsinger and colleagues (1979) performed an adoption study of suicide where he found that the biological relatives of 71 patients with affective disorder showed a 3.9% frequency of suicide. Adoptive relatives of these persons showed only .6% suicides, and adoptive relatives of control adoptees were similar to the adoptive relatives of the affectively ill probands. Mendlewicz and Rainer (1977) evaluated bipolar adoptees and found affective disorder in 31% of the biological parents of these probands compared with 2% in the biological parents of normal adoptees. The morbid risk for affective disorder in the biological parents was similar to the morbid risk in the parents of nonadopted bipolar patients (26%). Thus, there is clear evidence that a genetic factor is at work in the affective disorders and most particularly in bipolar affective disorder.

Finally, in bipolar illness, there is a possibility of linkage of a bipolar gene to markers on the X chromosome. However, not all findings have been positive, and this may be accounted for by the possibility of heterogeneity in the illness or an error due to simple chance. The first report of linkage with an X marker (color blindness) was published by Reich and associates (1969). Since that time, there have been a variety of positive and negative findings, including a positive study published by Baron and colleagues (1987) showing strong evidence of X linkage. However, in a reevaluation of the multigeneration kindred that Baron and co-workers reported, evidence for X linkage diminished in two of the families but remained positive in the third family (Baron et al. 1993).

In general then, good data exist to support a familial breeding true in schizophrenia as well as bipolar and unipolar illness. Most of these studies focus on individuals at a certain point in time, and no doubt in the course of the evolution of the illness some people will become ill that had previously been well. A particularly good methodology would be to take a group of probands, follow them prospectively until old age, and evaluate their siblings in particular, as they would have had exactly the same period of time in which to develop the illness.

# Chapter 5

# The Iowa 500

## *Genesis*

The starting flag for the Iowa 500 was dropped in late 1971 with the goal of collecting information that would advance the understanding of schizophrenia and the affective disorders, most specifically in relation to diagnostic validity, clinical features, course and outcome, and familial incidence. The study was designed to incorporate the most current research methodology. Originally, there was to be a systematic evaluation of clinical features and course of illness, a blind family interview, and a blind family history evaluation. But as we embarked on the study, we enlarged it to encompass a long-term personal examination of the probands and all of the relatives and to obtain comprehensive and standardized clinical and epidemiologic data using a structured interview. For the purpose of comparison and blindness, it became necessary to add to the 100 manic patients, the 225 depressive patients, and the 200 schizophrenic patients a control group that consisted of 160 nonpsychiatric patients who had been admitted to the surgical services of the University of Iowa Hospital for either an appendectomy or elective herniorrhaphy. Even at an early date, we were hoping to be able

41

to single out specific homogeneous disease entities and to offer valid criteria for these. We believed at the start that the groups of patients that we were studying constituted heterogeneous sets of illnesses.

The study was feasible because Iowa has a relatively stable population, and we didn't believe that patients would migrate outside of the state to any large extent. Migration within the state posed no problem as far as getting information was concerned. As mentioned in Chapter 1, to test the feasibility, social worker Barbara Norton attempted to locate the first 50 patients. Forty-nine were located, and information was available on the 50th. Thirty-six percent of the 50 were still alive, and 78% of those living were still living within Iowa. We estimated that based on these figures, 247 (35% of all the index patients and control subjects) were still living in or outside the state. We conservatively estimated that three first-degree relatives per family might be interviewed and that there would be about 2,500 relatives from whom we would be able to obtain clinical information. In fact, as time went on, we calculated that there were 4,094 first-degree relatives at the time of the follow-up who were age 18 or older who would be available for interviewing; we were able to trace 3,698 (90%). Of the 2,037 first-degree relatives who were alive, we were able to interview 1,578 or 77%.

During the 1930s and 1940s, the patients in this study had been admitted to the Iowa State Psychopathic Hospital, a 60-bed short-term treatment facility serving the entire state of Iowa. For each of the approximately 370 patients admitted annually, there was an original completely typewritten record of all psychiatric social service interviews, progress notes, laboratory studies, discharge summaries, and transcripts of interviews with the patients. We used research criteria to make the diagnoses from the records (Feighner et al. 1972), which were relatively objective, and to minimize the amount of clinical judgment needed in making a diagnosis. Also, their validity is supported by a large body of data from clinical follow-up and family studies. In fact, if one peruses the recent criteria that have been used for research and clinical work, it will be obvious that they bear similarities to the criteria that we used. We used the criteria for primary affective disorder, depressed type; primary affective disorder, manic type; and schizophrenia.

## Primary Affective Disorder, Depressed Type: A Through C Required

A. Dysphoric mood (depressed, sad)
B. At least four of the following:
   1. Anorexia or weight loss
   2. Sleep difficulty
   3. Loss of energy
   4. Agitation or retardation
   5. Loss of interest in usual activities (includes decreased libido)
   6. Self-reproach or guilt
   7. Diminished ability to think or concentrate
   8. Recurrent thoughts of death or suicide
C. At least a 1-month course before admission to hospital, without preexisting psychiatric illness

## Primary Affective Disorder, Manic Type: A Through C Required

A. Euphoria or irritability
B. At least two of the following:
   1. Hyperactivity
   2. Push of speech; pressure to keep on speaking
   3. Flight of ideas
   4. Grandiosity
   5. Decreased sleep
   6. Distractibility

C. At least a 2-week course before admission to hospital, without preexisting psychiatric illness

---

## Schizophrenia: A Through D Required

A. A chronic illness lasting at least 6 months before index hospital evaluation without return to premorbid level of psychosocial adjustment
B. Absence of affective symptoms sufficient to qualify for diagnosis of primary affective disorder
C. At least one of the following:
    1. Delusions or hallucinations in a clear sensorium
    2. Lack of logical or understandable verbal communication
D. At least two of the following:
    1. Single
    2. Poor premorbid social or work history
    3. Absence of alcoholism or drug abuse within 1 year of onset of psychosis
    4. Onset before 40 years of age
    5. Blunted affect

These criteria were altered slightly in that, for schizophrenia, the criterion, family history of schizophrenia, was replaced with blunted affect. This was done because we were going to embark on a family history study of psychiatric illness and we did not want the findings to be biased. Had we left the original criterion in, we would have loaded the sample with familial schizophrenia.

The original research criteria did not include blunted affect because it is almost always associated with psychosis (delusions and hallucinations) or incoherent verbal production. As abnormal affect has been a major symptom of schizophrenia, and as certain kinds of schizophrenia are mainly associated with blunted affect (simple schizophrenia, certain kinds of hebephrenic and catatonic schizophrenia), we believe that it deserved separate status as a criterion for schizophrenia.

New criteria that bear considerable relationship to each other have been published since the Feighner criteria (e.g., Research Diagnostic Criteria, DSM-III, DSM-III-R [American Psychiatric Association 1980, 1987]). Until this point, no empirical findings have shown any one criterion to be clearly superior to the others (Coryell and Zimmerman 1987).

For our study, a consecutive series of case records from the years 1935–1945 was reviewed and cases were included as part of the study if they met research criteria, regardless of the chart diagnosis. Follow-up information was available in the charts for most patients, but the assignment of patients to groups was done blindly to the knowledge of outcome. Although enough manic and depressive patients were collected from 1935 to the mid-1940s, only 174 schizophrenic patients could be collected through 1944; therefore, the series was completed from the year 1934 so that the length of follow-up would be appropriately long. The original chart diagnoses of the patients were based on the classification adopted by the American Psychiatric Association in 1934 (a Standard Classified Nomenclature of Disease, New York, Commonwealth Fund, 1933). For schizophrenia, subtype diagnosis was that of simple, hebephrenic, catatonic, or paranoid. A paranoid condition implied better preservation of affect and interests than seen in paranoid schizophrenia, which, in turn, was associated with better preservation of affect and interests than hebephrenic schizophrenia.

Concerning the behavior of the members of the psychiatric staff between 1934 and 1944, there were verbatim transcripts of staff meetings and interviews with the patients. These ran to as many as five single-spaced typewritten pages and reflected a vigorous debate, citation of facts from the psychiatric literature, minute examination of details of history or mental status, and considerable interpersonal heat. It was clear that diagnosis was of major importance during those years. Final diagnosis was arrived at by a vote of the attending and resident staff, and, when a differential diagnosis lay between an affective disorder and schizophrenia, preference was given to the former diagnosis. If the staff could not agree, the diagnosis was "undiagnosed."

About 3,800 patients were admitted to the hospital during the years covered by the study. At this time, about 13% of the patients were diagnosed as schizophrenic and 19% as having an affective disorder, manic depressive disease, or involutional melancholia (Morrison et al. 1972). We reviewed 874 charts of patients with affective psychoses and schizophrenia as well as innumerable charts with other diagnoses in order to obtain a sample of 525 patients. Table 5–1 presents the number of charts that were reviewed for each diagnosis and also the percentages that were discarded. Notably, though only one-quarter of the affective disorder charts were discarded, almost two-thirds of the charts of schizophrenic patients were dismissed from the study.

There were a variety of reasons for exclusion, as seen in Table 5–2. The modal reason for the exclusion of manic patients was the relatively short duration of symptoms; whereas, for depressed patients, the modal reason was the possibility of another diagnosis. This was also true for involutional melancholia. The schizophrenia criteria required at least 6 months of continuous illness and were, therefore, the major reason for eliminating schizophrenia charts. Of particular importance is the fact that 17% of patients with chart diagnoses of schizophrenia were excluded from the study because of an episodic course. The simple fact of having had an episodic course was

**Table 5–1.**  Charts reviewed to obtain 525 patients

| Chart diagnosis | Charts reviewed | Discarded (%) |
|---|---|---|
| Manic-depressive, manic type | 96 | 22 |
| Manic-depressive, depressed, or other manic-depressive types | 190 | 27 |
| Involutional melancholia | 84 | 20 |
| Schizophrenia | 504 | 63 |
| **Total** | **874** | |

*Source.*  Adapted from Morrison et al. 1972.

considered predictive of a future remitting or nonprocess course of the illness. A process course is one that terminates in a permanent thought disorder. All of these patients had already had a remission at some time prior to their discharge from their index hospitalization. Thirty-eight schizophrenic patients were eliminated because of insufficient symptoms. These patients had no delusions or hallucinations nor did they have any incoherence of speech. These were mainly simple schizophrenic patients. Most clinicians would probably agree that these patients suffered from schizophrenia, but, because they did not meet the criteria, they were removed from the study. The schizophrenic patients discarded from this project were later to become a very important subset of subjects for additional study. The reason there are relatively few catatonic subjects (2.5% of the schizophrenic patients) in the study is that they tended to have an acute onset and an episodic course and, therefore, had to be eliminated.

Patients in the affective disorder group were eliminated for the possibility of another diagnosis, and, to a large extent, this has to do with the presence of a secondary depression. Patients

**Table 5–2.** Reasons for excluding patients from follow-up and family study

| Reason for discard | Manic-depressive manic (*n* = 21) | Manic-depressive depressed (*n* = 51) | Involutional melancholia (*n* = 17) | Schizophrenia (*n* = 315) |
|---|---|---|---|---|
| Episodic course | 0 | 0 | 0 | 55 |
| Short duration of symptoms | 15 | 7 | 1 | 166 |
| Possibility of other diagnosis | 2 | 20 | 9 | 44 |
| Insufficient symptoms | 4 | 10 | 4 | 38 |
| IQ <70 only | 0 | 14 | 3 | 12 |

*Source.* Adapted from Morrison et al. 1972.

with hysteria, antisocial personality, or alcoholism may have depressions (secondary depressions) that are symptomatically indistinguishable from a primary depression, but these may differ markedly from primary depressions in course; thus, we chose only patients who suffered a primary depression. Primary depression is a depression that occurs in an individual who has had no other psychiatric illness except a prior episode of depression. A secondary depression is a depression that occurs after the onset of another psychiatric illness (i.e., antisocial personality, somatization disorder, alcoholism, schizophrenia, obsessive/compulsive disorder, agoraphobia, etc.).

Although follow-up information was available for most patients and was in the chart, the evaluators of the patients had no knowledge of the outcome until after each patient had been diagnosed and either included or excluded from the study. The follow-up material was in a separate part of the chart, and it was easy to keep the raters from seeing this material at the time of the diagnostic process. It was well recognized that the follow-up data might influence the diagnosis. Geographic factors may have also influenced severity as noted by the possibility that patients in close proximity to Iowa City might have had a less severe illness than patients farther away in Iowa, the former using hospitalization because of accessibility to some extent, the latter using it because of need. No data were recorded at the time of the beginning of the study to allow us to evaluate that possibility.

Table 5–3 presents the chart diagnoses of the final study groups. Reactive depressions were included under the group of manic-depressive depressed and differ from the other primary depressions in that they have a precipitating factor; however, we did not, in this study, consider that a reason for exclusion. In actuality, relatively few patients had a diagnosis of reactive depression. In the 1930s, most of the patients who were admitted were severely depressed, and, generally, reactive depressions are milder in nature than other kinds of depressions.

When the selection was complete, we had 200 schizophrenic, 100 manic (of whom 94 were manic at admission and six had a prior history of mania), and 225 depressive patients. Of those 225 depressive patients, a long follow-up of 30–40 years revealed that 22 of them (approximately 9%) had become bipolar. At time of admission, however, the characteristics of the patients chosen for the study appear in Table 5–4 (Clancy et al. 1974). Some marked differences existed among the groups. Whereas the schizophrenic patients were almost equally divided between the sexes, both the manic and the depressive patients show a female preponderance, which is greater in the group of manic patients. Schizophrenic patients were infrequently married and showed a high degree of poor premorbid adjustment and poor work history. However, as this symptom is a part of the criteria set for selection, the marked difference is not surprising. Only the depressive patients showed a large number of suicide attempts with the present illness, but, once again, this is a part of the selection criteria. We also found a significant differ-

**Table 5–3.**  Chart diagnoses in groups accepted for follow-up and family study

| Chart diagnosis | Unipolar affective disorder (n = 225) % | Bipolar affective disorder (n = 100) % | Schizophrenia (n = 200) % |
|---|---|---|---|
| Manic-depressive, depressed | 56.4 | 4.0 | 0 |
| Manic-depressive, manic | 0 | 75.0 | 0 |
| Other manic-depressive | 5.3 | 12.0 | 0 |
| Involutional melancholia | 29.9 | 0 | .5 |
| Simple schizophrenia | 0 | 1.0 | 7.0 |
| Paranoid schizophrenia | 0 | 0 | 27.5 |
| Hebephrenic schizophrenia | 0 | 0 | 35.0 |
| Catatonic schizophrenia | 0 | 1.0 | 2.5 |
| Other schizophrenia | 0 | 0 | 22.5 |
| Other diagnosis | 8.4 | 7.0 | 5.0 |

*Source.*  Adapted from Morrison et al. 1972.

**Table 5–4.**  Social and demographic characteristics of the Iowa
500 patients

| Characteristic | Schizophrenic (n = 200) n (%) | Manic (n = 100) n (%) | Depressive (n = 225) n (%) |
|---|---|---|---|
| Female | 97 (48.5) | 62 (62) | 125 (55.6) |
| Married | 40 (20) | 51 (51) | 166 (74) |
| Poor premorbid adjustment and work history | 100 (50) | 5 (5) | 7 (3) |
| High school graduate | 56 (28) | 29 (29) | 54 (24) |
| Suicide attempts with present illness | 2 (1) | 5 (5) | 61 (27) |
| Precipitating factors | 22 (11) | 27 (27) | 88 (39) |
| Age at onset (median) | 25.9 | 26.5 | 39.4 |
| Age at admission (median) | 27.0 | 30.1 | 44.8 |
| Ill more than 1 year before admission | 170 (85) | 11 (11) | 59 (26) |
| Discharged to community | 52 (26) | 39 (39) | 108 (48) |

*Source.*   Adapted from Clancy et al. 1974.

ence in precipitating factors between the schizophrenic and manic patients where the 2.5-fold difference in favor of the manic patients is significant at the .01 level of probability. What is particularly interesting is that the depressive patients have a significantly higher level of precipitating events than the manic patients ($P = .05$). The age at onset between the manic and schizophrenic patients is not notably different, but the depressive patients first become ill 13 years later than in both of these groups. The age at admission reflects this, and, in most of the studies that have been done, one can make a choice as to whether to use the age at onset or the age at admission. They are so clearly correlated that either one will separate groups.

Though the schizophrenic patients needed only to be ill 6 months prior to admission, 85% had been ill for more than 1 year. The manic patients, on the other hand, had been ill more than 1 year in only 11% of the cases, and this was less than one-half the amount of the depressive patients who had been ill for more than 1 year.

The discharge circumstances are of particular importance since, in the days of these admissions, there was no treatment. Nevertheless, almost half of the depressive patients and 40% of the manic patients were discharged from the hospital to the community, but this occurred in only one-quarter of the schizophrenic patients.

As noted before, the charts were complete enough so that it was possible to have follow-up data on almost all of the patients. On the average, patients were followed for several years by social workers who sent out letters to the families. In fact, some patients were followed-up for as many as 20–40 years, while others had very short follow-up periods. The social workers also collected a systematic family history, which was recorded in the chart. All information was often supplemented by material from the residents and staff psychiatrists. The next step in the Iowa 500 was to evaluate the follow-up material and the family history material from the charts, but prior to that we will present some of the verbatim interviews with the patients.

# Chapter 6

# Real People

## *Histories and Verbatim Interviews*

Neither the quality of the patient nor the quality of the illness is well conveyed by numbers and tables. Even a narrative, though a considerable improvement over the simple presentation of numbers, may leave something to be desired. However, if we can capture a real person by presenting his or her feelings and thoughts and behavior in the individual's own words, we can come closer to our understanding of both the person and the illness. Descriptions, interviews, and staff discussions follow about patients who had depression, mania, or schizophrenia at the time of admission to the Iowa Psychopathic Hospital. These patients are part of the group that was chosen for the Iowa 500. They are typical of patients that were seen then and are seen now.

These interviews were recorded verbatim by a secretary at the time they occurred. They are presented in their original form, warts and all.

On reading some of the interviews, people have noted that, unlike the current popular interview style, the physician often asked leading questions. No attempt was made by the examiner to present an open-ended situation in which the patient was encouraged to express himself or herself in an ordinary conversational way. The reason for this is clear. The physicians were attempting to assess the clinical state of the patient in an organized fashion. By the time of interview, the physicians knew a great deal about the patients, or, if they interviewed the patient late in the hospitalization, they were particularly interested in assessing change and the presence or absence of clinical symptomatology that had been present at admission. Thus, the goal of the interview was to assess the clinical state of the patient and the state of the patient's illness. The goal was not to provide an open field for the expression of concerns or problems of daily living.

The *dramatis personae* were as follows: Dr. Andrew Woods, professor and head of the department of psychiatry, University of Iowa, and director of the Iowa Psychopathic Hospital. The supporting physicians included the following: Dr. Walter Thompson, who was a resident at the time of the interview and later became assistant clinical professor of psychiatry at Tulane University and Baylor University; Dr. William Malamud, who was a member of the faculty and became professor and chairman at Boston University; Dr. J. Franklin Robinson, a resident who became the senior chief of the psychiatric service at the Wilkes-Barre General Hospital in Pennsylvania; Dr. Jacques Gottlieb, who was a resident and became professor and chairman of Wayne State University in Detroit; Dr. Cyril Ruilman, who was a resident and became associate professor at Meharry Medical College and Vanderbilt University Medical School; Dr. Hale Shirley, a member of the faculty who became professor of psychiatry and pediatrics at Stanford University; Dr. I. Paley Rubin, who was a resident; Dr. Rex Buxton, who was a resident and became a training analyst at the Washington Psychoanalytic Institute; Dr. Isadore Rodis, a resident who became clinical professor of psychiatry at Georgetown University; Dr. Erich Lindeman, a member of the faculty who became professor of psychiatry at Harvard University; Dr. William Orr, a resident who became professor and department head at Vanderbilt University; Dr. Wilbur Miller, a member of the faculty who became professor and head of the department at the University of Iowa; Dr. Lois Lobb, a resident who became a private practitioner; Dr. Harold Lovell, a member of the faculty who became clinical professor of neurology at New York Medical College; Dr. Howard Weatherly, a resident who became assistant clinical professor of psychiatry at UCLA; and Dr. Marcus Emmons, a resident who went into private practice in Iowa and was the past president of the Iowa Psychiatric Association.

## The Depressive Patients

### ▎ CHD

A 55-year-old married policeman was admitted September 23, 1937. For 7 months, he had been despondent with thoughts of and attempts at suicide. He thought people were after him and that he had done something for which he would be sent to the state penitentiary. He became restless, frightened, and tried to hide himself. He had shot himself in the city hall several months before in a fit of despair over the noise of children and dogs. The bullet was still lodged in his brain, and he had three epileptiform fits. However, his despondency increased with threats of suicide and "taking his wife with him" until the family was finally frightened enough to have him hospitalized.

At the time of admission, he appeared a solemn, gaunt man. He lay on the cot and was cooperative, but bewildered, and retarded with his speech. He left his sentences unfinished. He said that he was "crooked" as a law officer and had been trying to tell his family but they wouldn't listen. He seemed unable to accomplish the ordinary sensorium tests because of lack of attention and comprehension, depression and retardation of motor activity and speech, defective memory, and ideas of self-depreciation and being discriminated against. He had trouble concentrating and lacked any kind of insight or judgment.

Past history was significant in that, at age 33, he had a

failure in business and had a nervous breakdown during which time he was despondent for 6 months. His normal personality was that of a calm and resourceful person, reserved, but probably overly conscientious. The day after admission, he was seen in ward rounds in the morning and was interviewed by Dr. Andrew Woods.

Q:  How is this kind of weather to you? [Raining]
A:  (Long pause) Not so good.
Q:  Do you always feel blue on rainy days?
A:  (Pause) Well, not necessarily.
Q:  What makes you feel bad?
A:  (No answer)

He remained in the hospital until October 14, 1937, and, prior to discharge, he was interviewed by Dr. Woods at a staff meeting. The interview follows:

Q:  What do you feel like doing today?
A:  Well, I am not sure, for certain.
Q:  Would it be nice to go outside and take a walk or do some work?
A:  (Nods head yes)
Q:  You were working at a coal mine, were you, recently?
A:  I had been before I came up here.
Q:  Have you a job open to you still?
A:  No, I don't think so; they don't have many jobs for men of 55 or more.
Q:  But you had a job before you came here?
A:  Yes.
Q:  Why isn't it open to you now?
A:  It seems as though the mines have cut off men of this age.
Q:  Did you get any word of that?
A:  I heard it hinted I was out of a job.
Q:  There are men older than 55 who are working?
A:  Yes, but they had work before this ruling started.
Q:  How did you learn of it?
A:  I got it up there at the union meeting.

**Q:**  Before you came here?

**A:**  Uh-huh.

**Q:**  If you don't go back to mine work, what would you like to do?

**A:**  Well, I would like to do anything I could get to do, if I don't go back to the mine.

**Q:**  You are well and strong and capable of working. Is there any reason to fear you will not get a job?

**A:**  No, I suppose not.

**Q:**  When you came here, did you want to get help about something? Were you sick in some way?

**A:**  Well, I understood from some of my folks that they had me sent up here.

**Q:**  Why was that?

**A:**  I suppose there was a reason of some kind.

**Q:**  What do you think the reason was?

**A:**  Well, my daughter, she seems to think if I write home, everything will be all right. Well, I don't know whether it will be or not.

**Q:**  Was it your daughter who brought you here?

**A:**  One of my daughters.

**Q:**  What do you think was in her mind? Was she trying to help you or hurt you?

**A:**  Well, I don't think she has got all in her mind she ought to have before she come.

**Q:**  What was the reason she wanted to bring you here?

**A:**  She has got a husband up there in Des Moines and he is crippled up in his back a little now, and I have an idea if I write back saying what I suspect why he will try to slip out easy.

**Q:**  What is it you suspect?

**A:**  Well, (pause) I think he thinks I never will come back.

**Q:**  Can you tell me why it was your daughter brought you up here?

**A:**  I suppose (long pause) she wants to hold on to her man; I can't think of anything else.

**Q:**  Why should she bring you up here in order to hold on to her man?

A:  Well, I know I was.

Q:  What do you think was the reason why she brought you here? Did it have any connection with you?

A:  (Pause) The only thing I can think of that was anything like that was Jim made a threat one time if I had dirty feet I could beat him, see?

Q:  Did that have anything to do with her bringing you here?

A:  I don't know.

Q:  What could it have had to do? Do you think your daughter and your friends wanted to help you when they brought you here or were they trying to injure you?

A:  It seems as though they meant to help me.

Q:  What did they want to help you for? What was the matter?

A:  (Pause) Well, I don't know what it would be unless they could start something of that kind. I don't know what else.

Q:  Have you in the last 4 or 5 years done anything that was crooked?

A:  Well, (pause) right now I can't think of anything I have done that was straight.

Q:  How is it all of your friends speak very highly of you; they say you have been an honest man and a good husband and father.

A:  I don't know unless it is just an exceeding exception to say it is.

Q:  What is that?

A:  Unless it is an exceedingly big discrepancy, I don't know.

Q:  Can you tell me any one thing you have done to make people distrust you?

A:  (No answer)

Q:  You have not hurt anyone; you have not stolen anything. What is there they could blame you for?

A:  Well, there might be several little places that don't look so bad, but if you pinched them up together, it looks bad enough.

**Q:** Have you noticed people looking at you in any unusual way as if they were blaming you?

**A:** No, not lately I haven't.

**Q:** What did you notice previously?

**A:** Well, in the last month or so I noticed several odd, stiff-necked people when I spoke to them.

**Q:** While here in the hospital, have the doctors and nurses and other patients been that way?

**A:** Well, I don't know as they have.

**Q:** They all seem to like you, don't they?

**A:** Yes.

**Q:** If you are such a bad man, how does it come they like you?

**A:** I don't know.

**Q:** Do you really think you are a bad man?

**A:** Coming right down to final details, I don't think I am a bad man.

**Q:** Do you think they really believe you are a bad man?

**A:** I think they think more like that than anything else.

**Q:** While you have been here, have you heard them talking about you?

**A:** No.

**Q:** Have you seen people pointing at you as if they were talking about you?

**A:** No.

**Q:** And at night in your bed when it is quiet, do you ever hear people saying things about you or hear the radio talking about you?

**A:** I can hear the radio all the time when I'm home.

**Q:** Do you hear it talking about you?

**A:** Oh, no.

**Q:** At night, do you ever hear people talking as if they were talking about you?

**A:** (Pause) Well, one time I made the remark to my son-in-law that the only thing my wife listened to was the local news and that is about all she listens to, you know.

**Q:** But that had nothing to do with your reputation.

**A:** No more than just murders, something like that.

Q: As you look forward to next year, what do you think your chances are to get work and get back into your life?

A: (Pause) Well, I suppose—you know—I don't know whether I can prove Mrs. B was carrying my bond or not.

Q: You were under bond for what purpose.

A: Marshal.

Q: Are you the town marshal?

A: Yes.

Q: You had to give a bond for that.

A: Yes.

Q: That bond doesn't act on you unless you do something wrong, so looking forward to next year, there is nothing to interfere about the bond?

A: I wouldn't think so. It looks to me like if they were going to do anything about filing my bond, it would have started before this.

Q: As to working, do you feel there is good hope you will get back into work?

A: It all depends. You see, I hauled shale on the streets last year, and, at first, I never thought about getting the approval of my councilmen.

Q: That's all past. We won't talk about that. As to getting a new job and getting started again, why should you not go right ahead?

A: I don't know that I have a reason for not going ahead.

Q: Do you feel hopeful about it?

A: Yes.

Q: You would like to go back home then and get started into work and take care of your family?

A: If I could.

Q: Why shouldn't you?

A: Because some other guys wouldn't let me is all I know.

Q: Wouldn't let you do what?

A: Take another job.

Q: Suppose you were to get sick now, rather seriously sick, as you lay in bed, would you like to think of get-

ting well and going back home or would you rather
not live through it?

A: Well, if things were so back home like they used to
be, I would like to be there.

Q: As they actually are now, would you rather live on
and get back into life again?

A: I wouldn't mind if it was so I could.

Q: What do you think about it?

A: I believe I could.

The patient was sent on to a state hospital for further care
with the diagnosis of manic-depressive psychosis, depressed.

His family history was positive. His youngest sister had
manic-depressive illness, and a nephew of the patient was
in the state hospital for a short time because of "overex-
haustion." He recovered.

There was no short-term follow-up on this man in that he
had gone to one of the state hospitals that did not cooper-
ate in providing follow-up information.

## ▌ LBD

LBD was a 34-year-old single factory worker who had been
working steadily for the past 19 years making feather dust-
ers. She was admitted in the late part of November 1938
after losing interest in her work 3 months earlier. For
2 weeks, she had been very depressed and despondent and
felt that she had a bad disease. When admitted, she had
been malnourished, agitated, and withdrawn. She refused
to answer questions about her feelings.

Her family history was positive; her father had experienced a period of "melancholy" that had lasted 4–6 months
when he was about 45 years old. This was supposed to have
been due to financial worries. Her mother, in her late 50s,
had a mild depressive period that lasted for 6 months; however, she was able to continue to work. None of the siblings
had any illness.

On admission, a mental status conducted on November 25 revealed that she talked distinctly, refused to express her feelings, and was mute in response to questions about her present illness, but she would respond promptly to questions concerning her past history. She seemed on the verge of tears and, at times, became agitated. It was felt that her mood was that of deep depression. She felt strong guilt, which was related to delusions that she had a venereal disease. There was no evidence of bizarre associations, but her memory and sensorium appeared to be impaired by her mood.

Her course in the hospital a few days after admission revealed little change. She lay in bed with the sheets pulled up around her mouth and mumbled her answers. In early December, she had a few changes in her thought content, namely some ideas of reference. At times, she seemed almost bright and happy; however, by December 13th, it was noted that she had continued to lose weight and her mental status was unchanged. She slept poorly and was considered deeply depressed, and occasionally she refused to talk. She was agitated and fearful.

On December 23, 1938, the patient was interviewed by Dr. Woods, and the following interview was presented:


Q:　It is a nice bright day out, isn't it?

A:　(No answer)

Q:　Does it make you feel better when you see the sun shining?

A:　(No answer)

Q:　Have you noticed that all the women in the ward are getting ready for Christmas?

A:　(No answer)

Q:　When you don't answer questions, is it because you don't feel friendly to us, or are you angry at us?

A:　(No answer)

Q:　Can you tell me?

A:　(No answer)

Q:　Would you like to go away leaving the impression you didn't like us and didn't want to talk to us?

A:　(No answer)

**Q:** I would like to know if you feel friendly to us or not.

**A:** (No answer)

**Q:** If it is hard to talk, suppose you nod your head if you do feel friendly to us.

**A:** (No response of any kind)

**Q:** Have we tried to be good to you?

**A:** (No answer)

**Q:** All right, we won't trouble you any more. You can go back to the ward.

In the staff conference following that interview, the diagnosis of "manic-depressive, depressed" was given to the patient. (In the 1930s, all patients with affective psychoses were diagnosed as "manic-depressive.") There was some question about the depression being "involutional" though all agreed that they would not want to call it involutional as there was "no involution." The staff agreed that she had not improved and, in fact, was worse, and they decided to administer Metrazol treatments. The patient appeared to improve somewhat after the seventh injection of Metrazol (six convulsions in all). By the end of January she was definitely brighter. However, after the treatments had been stopped, she became more agitated. She was transferred to a state hospital.

The follow-up was interesting. She was admitted to the state hospital in April 1939 and discharged as cured April 8, 1940. She was considered completely recovered.

## ∎ RHD

A 23-year-old single man was referred from neurology because of complaints of depression, loss of interest, restlessness, and a suicide attempt. Though admitted July 5, 1937, he had been depressed since January of that year. Before admission, he had talked about suicide and made an attempt in the latter part of June by putting a rope around his neck.

The informants believed there was a change in the patient's general behavior 2 years prior to admission. At that time, it was felt that he was becoming overly ambitious and made plans that were not in line with his former behavior. It is conceivable that he was hypomanic. In January, he was jilted by a girl, and the depressive episode that led to the index admission started about then.

The records include two, single-spaced, typewritten pages on the family history, and there were no first-degree relatives or extended relatives considered as having had a psychiatric illness. After staying a short time in the hospital, he was discharged on August 16, the day before, he was interviewed by Dr. Woods.

Q: Are you feeling fine this morning?
A: Pretty good.
Q: Do you feel like going back to work?
A: Yes.
Q: How long has it been since you really felt like working?
A: Oh, about 4 weeks.
Q: When was it you left your mother's place to take up work of your own?
A: I left my mother—well, I stayed there most of the time, see, and worked away from home.
Q: When did you take a farm outside?
A: In March.
Q: Of this year?
A: Yes.
Q: Didn't you try farming in the year 1936?
A: Yes.
Q: That was the time you left your mother's place to work for yourself?
A: Yes. I tried to farm in 1937.
Q: When you took a farm for yourself, were you feeling quite well? Did you feel you could make a success?
A: I thought I could.
Q: What happened? Did you continue to feel you could do it?
A: I got discouraged.
Q: That was early in 1937?

**A:** Yes, I went all to pieces.

**Q:** Do you remember how you felt at that time? Did you feel sick or weak?

**A:** I was discouraged because my plans fell through.

**Q:** What does that mean?

**A:** I thought I used poor judgment.

**Q:** When you took the farm in 1937, you became discouraged because you thought you had used poor judgment?

**A:** Yes.

**Q:** As you look back, do you feel that you did use poor judgment?

**A:** I don't believe I did.

**Q:** If you had the same sort of opening, could you make a success of it?

**A:** I believe so.

**Q:** What seems to be the difference? Why should you have been discouraged?

**A:** I don't know. Everything was awfully high at that time.

**Q:** Did the feeling of discouragement come on quickly?

**A:** The realization that I didn't really need a farm was the trouble.

**Q:** You felt you should have stayed at your mother's place?

**A:** Yes.

**Q:** But wasn't it wisest for you to start out for yourself?

**A:** I suppose.

**Q:** Was it too big a farm?

**A:** It was too large an undertaking.

**Q:** But if you had it now, could you make a success of it?

**A:** I think so.

**Q:** What would you like to do now?

**A:** Go home and farm.

**Q:** Do you feel now that if you had a farm of your own, you could be successful?

**A:** I believe I could.

**Q:** What sort of farm would you want? How would it be different from your first one?

A: I would want improvements on it.

Q: Had you thought of getting married when you went out for yourself?

A: Yes, I thought about getting married some time in the future.

Q: Was there some particular girl?

A: Yes.

Q: What happened about that?

A: It became best not to go together at that time.

Q: Was that because she had changed?

A: I wanted to find out something about her.

Q: Did you mean there was something possibly wrong with her?

A: Yes.

Q: Was that something you discovered only after you made the change about the farm?

A: Yes.

Q: Is it something you can talk about? What was the reason you felt there might be something wrong with her? Was it about her health or character?

A: Health.

Q: What do you think of her now?

A: I think she is a nice woman.

Q: Has she married in the meantime?

A: Yes.

Q: Do you feel now that the doubt you had about her was not well founded?

A: I am undetermined.

Q: You haven't made up your mind about that yet?

A: Sometimes I think I am wrong.

Q: Do you regret having given her up?

A: Yes, in a way I do.

Q: You have some other women friends?

A: I have several since then.

Q: Was your family and friends kind to you about this venture of yours? Did they try to help you?

A: Yes.

Q: Do you feel that with their help, you might be able to succeed if you had gone on?

**A:**  I should have been able to.

**Q:**  How are you sleeping now?

**A:**  Nothing extraordinary.

**Q:**  Do you worry in the night when you are awake?

**A:**  Sometimes.

**Q:**  During the day time, do you keep thinking about these things and worrying over them?

**A:**  Yes.

**Q:**  When you do worry now, what things trouble you?

**A:**  I worry about being placed like this.

**Q:**  Why does that worry you?

**A:**  I think I should be home.

**Q:**  Do you feel you are just as capable now as you were?

**A:**  Yes, I am as strong.

**Q:**  How about the worry and discouragement—could you make a success of it worrying as much as you are now?

**A:**  (No answer)

**Q:**  Suppose you were at home this morning, would you feel like going out and starting work?

**A:**  Yes.


**Dr. Woods:**  Dr. Robinson suggests that the patient seems to be discouraged and downcast, and that he is manic-depressive, depressed. Is that satisfactory? (All agree.)

**Dr. Robinson:**  He talked this morning about the same way in which he talked when he came in. For a couple of weeks he looked better. There was one instance when he was on convalescent ward and then was moved back to receiving when he was very depressed.

**Dr. Woods:**  Is there any difference in the course of the day?

**Dr. Robinson:**  In the day time he seems much better. He has been playing with two youngsters on the ward. There is not much difference during the day.

**Dr. Woods:**  Dr. Malamud, do you feel he would be safe in the care of relatives?

**Dr. Malamud:**   I wonder if he would be any safer now
than when he first came in, although I don't know
that there was danger even then. This morning, I
don't see much change from when I talked to him
when I left. There seems to be a great deal under the
surface which we have not reached yet. His slowness
looks more like preoccupation than the retardation
usually seen in manic depressives. I think that there
will be difficulty if he goes out but on the other
hand, I think he should be tried. I would suggest
that he be paroled to the care of one of his relatives.
He could come back in a month or 6 weeks at which
time we could see.

He was discharged against medical advice and went home,
but it was the general impression of the people in the hospital that he should be followed. On November 30, 1938,
his sister wrote that he was still not quite as well as the
family would like, though he had improved. By March of
1939, his sister said that he was quite a bit better, was taking more interest in his surroundings, and enjoying social-
izing with young people. He was interested in seeking some
kind of employment. The case was closed in June 1939.

---

## The Manic Patients

### ▎ IPM

A 38-year-old woman was admitted May 9, 1935. She was excited, talked constantly, and expressed many irrelevant ideas,
and it was almost impossible to carry on a conversation with
her. Her husband had died about 2 weeks earlier, and, at his
funeral, she became excited and overtalkative. Her mental
status conducted on the day of admission follows:

**Patient:**   Well, they think I'm nuts. I'm not nuts. If I
make a pledge I stick to it through thick and thin.

I married for love not for money. Somebody is playing a dirty trick on me. I'll kick him right out of the
state. You know who they are. How many names have
you there? If he were to die I would kick him and enjoy it. There was a blonde there and they said what
kind of a show we were running. I could face him
face to face. I got some friends someplace. There
were two lives lost in Marengo on the City Council.
John Pater lies and lies. Gip, Gip, Gibson was the old
fellow there. They don't want to break up their
home. They won't do that. I got a new permanent.
You know when I got it?

**Q:** Are you sick?

**A:** No I feel fine. I'm just flipsy flopsy. It isn't the truth
that hurts, it is just lies, lies.

**Q:** Do you usually talk this way?

**A:** No.

**Q:** Why do you do it now?

**A:** Well, my mind is an open book. What was his was
mine, what was mine was his. Now he is gone.
I wouldn't ask him to come back. I keep my pledge.
You will keep yours, won't you? If they need to be
punished, I'm not guilty. Ask Dr. L. I swabbed out his
ear and got water in mine.

**Q:** Why do you feel this way?

**A:** Because I've been accused of that all my life.

**Q:** Accused of what?

**A:** Oh, I don't know. I have been accused of this and accused of that.

**Q:** What were you accused of?

**A:** Well, they said I pay for them. She married that big
hog, brazen Raines.

**Q:** Who?

**A:** Dr. Raines.

**Q:** Why call him a hog?

**A:** He said I paid him and paid him and if I changed—oh
dear, I'm getting so weak. I said it so many times.

**Q:** What do you mean?

**A:** He said if I tried everything he tried it would be too

late. He was from Chicago. He was one of those wise
guys who ought to go back and get some more training. He can walk the straight and narrow from now
on. One, two, three. I can't shed anymore tears. I've
shed so many tears I can't cry anymore. They
thought I was crazy. I was friendly, I like to talk to
people. That big brazen hog, I would stick him if you
gave me a pitchfork. I didn't want but one man. Do
you believe me? My father stuck to me through thick
and thin. My mother is dead. Please let her rest.
Don't go back that far. Oh my, my, my, my, my. I just
wanted one man (cries hard).

Her past history was negative for any prior illness. She had
no medical problems. Her course in the hospital was re-
markable because of the fact that, for the first 3 weeks of
her stay there, her behavior and stream of talk and thought
was typical of a manic psychosis. She was excited, laughed,
cried, alternately yelled, and talked continuously. Associations were rapid. It was necessary to sedate her with cold,
wet sheet packs and sedatives. After 3 weeks, the episodes
subsided, and she became overly affectionate and cheerful,
though, on occasion, tearful. She still showed some residual, emotional lability at discharge. An interview with one
of the members of the staff, Dr. Shirley, on May 23 follows.
(The patient still showed some flight of ideas.) She was discharged on June 18, 1935, to her home environment under
the supervision of her father. Her last interview, which is
presented verbatim, was performed by Dr. Woods on the day
of her discharge. There was no disagreement about diagnosis after the interview by Dr. Woods, although the staff did
think that she was not totally well. There is no short-term
follow-up in the chart.

## May 23, 1935

A:　You are not going to play any tricks on me, are you?
Q:　No. How are you feeling?
A:　My feelings is all right.
Q:　What are you crying about?

A: Well, that's my business.

Q: Tell me.

A: I know who you are.

Q: Tell me.

A: Mr. Van Epps, aren't you?

Q: Have you been sick?

A: No.

Q: Have you been acting peculiarly?

A: No, they have been acting peculiar with me and I guess I should-a showed them how it was too.

Q: What?

A: Well, that's the trouble and nobody knows our troubles. That was out of the eyes, out of this and out of that but that was all inside of the family but people never did.

Q: What?

A: Well, that's it. No use to tell it now.

Q: What has been troubling you?

A: Well, I'll never tell. I was crushing my father and then my mother died.

Q: What do you mean?

A: Well, if I tell you the whole world will know. I better not.

Q: What was this about crushing your father?

A: I never told him about any of my troubles. He's still living isn't he? He should be. What is today?

Q: What is it?

A: Well, I don't know. They keep telling me the same day all the time.

Q: What month is this?

A: May, I think. June, July, August, September, I don't know what month it is. Did you ever know anybody who'd marry for a hundred thousand dollars and not marry for love? Well, I did. I took the M name and I'm proud of it. When it was his side of the house, it was doctah, doctah, doctah this and doctah that and when it came to me, I was the dirt on the steps and Otto, oh, no. Otto wasn't the dirt on the steps but I had that from the family, the M family all my life.

Q: Have the Ps mistreated you? Hmm?

A: Oh, I don't know. It's got too late now. Otto's gone. Otto R. M. He's my husband. I'm proud of it. I wish you all to know I'm proud of it but he's gone now. I'm still here. I guess I'm here. You know that. And as long as you can work and work. I have still got the sewing machine. I'm out . . . (indistinct) went to Burlington, Iowa, on their honeymoon and got their furniture and we got ours.

Q: How do they treat you here in the hospital?

A: Well, that's it. I don't belong here in this part because I never told anybody of my troubles. Who brought me down here, do you know?

Q: Tell me what your troubles are.

A: Who brought me down here, that's what I ask.

Q: What are your troubles?

A: I haven't any troubles.

Q: Who is trying to hurt you?

A: Well, I'm not crazy. I haven't lost my mind. Well, you are the doctor, aren't you?

Q: Have they been putting poison in your food?

A: Well, I don't know. They tell me this and they tell me that, and I can't get to the telephone to get to the doctor that I know. I know who you are. I have seen you lots of times when I passed your office. I'm not crazy.

## June 18, 1935

Q: Do you feel quite cheerful today?

A: Yes, sir.

Q: Have you had a good time in this hospital?

A: Yes, I had a good time since I found out where I was.

Q: Was it hard to know where you were?

A: Yes, at first.

Q: You could ask anybody?

A: Yes, I could, but I didn't.

Q: Where did you think you were?

A: I thought I was in—

Q: Didn't you realize where you were?

A: I don't know, several weeks ago.

Q: Do you remember the first week or 10 days you were here?

A: I remember some.

Q: What were you doing?

A: Talking. I couldn't stop, I guess.

Q: Do you think you talked more than usual?

A: Yes, sir.

Q: Why did you do that?

A: I think I became hysterical and talked and cried.

Q: Do you remember making an effort to stop talking?

A: No, it seemed like I couldn't.

Q: Did you try to stop?

A: No. I thought there were so many strangers, and then I found that Miss Van Vessen was really a nurse.

Q: Can you remember how you felt during that first week? Did you feel angry at us, or happy, or how did you feel?

A: I couldn't control myself, I guess.

Q: Were you afraid of something?

A: I grieved over the loss of my husband, I guess.

Q: You had been doing that before.

A: Yes.

Q: But when you came here you were talking a great deal and behaving in a queer way. Do you remember how you felt that made you do that?

A: (No answer)

Q: Did you feel angry at us for having you here?

A: No, sir.

Q: How many days or weeks ago was it that you felt at home here and enjoyed being here?

A: When I was in the first ward a little over a week, I thought the nurses were all fine and the doctors. I've been here about 6 weeks altogether.

Q: Can you remember feeling different from the way you felt before?

A: Yes, sir.

Q: Are you sleeping better now than you did at first?

A:  Yes, sir.

Q:  Do you dream at night?

A:  No.

Q:  Do you remember that they gave you packs rather often.

A:  Yes, sir.

Q:  What did you make out of that? At the time, did you think it was good for you or how did you feel about it?

A:  I thought it was kind of ornery, and I couldn't help myself.

Q:  Did it make you mad when they put you in packs?

A:  Not after they told me it was good for me. I didn't understand at first.

Q:  Don't you think it would be a good plan for you to go back to your father and get to feeling completely well?

A:  Everything is clear now, and I understand things.

Q:  You are still nervous and shaky. You ought to be in a quiet place for a while where there is someone to look after you.

A:  I have plenty to look after me, my relatives at home.

Q:  Do you mean your father's home?

A:  I have a home of my own.

Q:  Where you and your husband lived?

A:  Yes, sir (patient cries).

Q:  Who is there to take care of you?

A:  My nephew and his wife.

Q:  Do you like them very much?

A:  Yes, sir.

Q:  They are good to you?

A:  Yes.

Q:  You will be shaky for a while so you ought to go back gradually to your ordinary work. All right, that will be all this morning. The diagnosis for this patient was manic-depressive psychosis, manic type.

## ▊ AFM

A 56-year-old woman was admitted December 20, 1937. She had experienced a mental illness of a "periodic" type for over 20 years, and, during the past 10 years, the intervals between the attacks had become increasingly brief. Her difficulty started at age 32, about a year after the birth of her first child. She became excitable and was hospitalized. After several months, she returned home and remained well for about 5 years when she had a second attack. She was again hospitalized and, since that time, had attacks that were described as periods of mild excitement ranging to periods of extreme overactivity and overtalkativeness with many bizarre ideas and periods of depression regressing to a level of stupor. In the past 2 years, she had been hospitalized for 18 of the 24 months.

When seen in the hospital, her associations were frequently of the clang variety. She had many bizarre ideas and spoke of alien control, hypnotism, and mental telepathy. A staff meeting was held 7 days after her admission, which was also the day that she was discharged to go to another hospital. It was noted that she had remained in the hospital for only 7 days, and there was no change in her mental status during this period.

At the hospital to which she was referred, not much change was observed in the patient. The statement was "her general mental condition of a hallucinatory nature remains with her." This was March 1938. By June 1938, the same hospital noted "she has improved greatly and has not recently had any spells of excitement." In January 1939, she was much improved and was allowed to go to town alone; there were no signs of deterioration.

## December 27, 1937

Q: Do you find it pleasant to live in the hospital?
A: Much more pleasant than where I have been.
Q: Where would you like to go to live?
A: I would prefer to go home or to be near one of my children.
Q: Who would be at your home?
A: No one, but I might find someone to live with me.
Q: Do you own your home?

A: I do.

Q: It would be available?

A: Yes, it is empty at present.

Q: When did you lose your husband?

A: He died the 13th of August of this year.

Q: Was his death sudden?

A: It was. He had apoplexy. He had a stroke the 9th of August in St. Louis and died the 15th, which was on Friday.

Q: You have always been a great reader?

A: Yes, I have read quite a lot.

Q: After you finished high school, did you go to college?

A: I went to what they called a practice or model school. The summer I was 14 I entered college. I was quite small for my age and the president said to me, "Why don't you go down stairs where you belong?" We were allowed to go from the 8th grade to college after we had one year of preparation.

Q: What kind of literature do you enjoy most?

A: Oh, I have read all kinds.

Q: Do you enjoy scientific literature?

A: Yes I do. About telepathy and hypnotism I have tried to find out what I could.

Q: You have had experience enough so you know about it?

A: I have.

Q: What kind of experiences have you had?

A: I will give you an example. Two years ago I was in the hospital. I was quite nervous at the time, and my brother and husband asked me to go to Chicago and consult a doctor who was a psychologist. I was quite uneasy because I had been down at Keokuk and I felt I would not like for us to take part in making arrangements for anyone else to go there. That night, I was praying that we might be able to help this man and keep him out of the place. I did not want anyone else to go through what I have. I feel that through telepathy he was able to contact my thoughts in that direction and that naturally it might happen; just as two wires cross so might our thoughts cross. It wasn't a work language but a thought language.

Q: Could you distinguish that from a thought which happened to come into your mind?

A: Yes. I had another experience with Fred S. His cousin's husband had died. She had been in a sanitarium in Macon. He had begged her husband to let her come out. He said she would be much better out of the place and she died. That night he died. Someone phoned me that Paul H. had died, so I told Mr. F. (husband) I would like to go down there. It seemed that someone said to me "Are you afraid? Are you afraid?" It seemed to me that I was being directed and it seemed to be her husband who was at the— Oh, you don't call it the morgue—the mortuary.

Q: While you have been here, have you been able to think about these things and get further experiences?

A: I feel that I have had things verified for me. For instance, you came into the hall the other day and I noticed that your chain did not have a charm on it. I had been thinking of charms and I felt that you were verifying something. There have been one or two other verifications that have come to me. For instance, as one gentleman came in, he nodded to me and I thought he was verifying that he had my thought. I think there has been enough so that part of it is true.

Q: How can you distinguish a thought that may come into your mind and one that comes from someone else?

A: I have presented several sides of the question to myself.

Q: Is it ever as distinct as a voice?

A: Once or twice. However, the quality of the voice is a little different. For instance, I had been thinking a great deal of my husband, and one morning I had the idea that he might come here. I had the thought that he was going into the garden and was calling me to see something in the garden.

Q:  Is there ever any visual confirmation of it? Do you
    see things that are extraordinary?

A:  I often see a resemblance in people. For instance, af-
    ter my father died, one day I saw a clear resemblance
    to him in another man which quickly disappeared.

Q:  Have you ever had any extraordinary visual phenom-
    ena? Have you seen things which you felt confirmed
    these ideas?

A:  I think I have. I have had unrelated ideas that were
    unimportant but later when they would tie them-
    selves together, they were important. For instance,
    the man who interrogated me a while back spoke
    aside to one or two of the men. I wondered what
    terms he was using. I thought they must be psycho-
    logical, and I got the idea that he said there was no
    set pattern but I felt there was a pattern.

Q:  You have been in various hospitals during the past
    25 years. Has there been any reason for this?

A:  There have been shocks.

Q:  Of what nature?

A:  The first was when my daughter began walking and
    burned her hands on the gas stove. The flesh was
    burned and you could see the bones. I knew of her
    agony and suffered with her. Later, because I was not
    kept busy, I had a breakdown.

Q:  In the breakdown, what did you experience? What
    changes went on?

A:  I was very fearful that something would happen to
    Mr. F. and when they divided my children among my
    sisters and others, I was uneasy about them being
    away. I thought that something might happen to
    Mr. F. and that I might die and he could not come.

Q:  Do you consider your nervousness as being a mental
    disease?

A:  I would think of it as a mental disease.

Q:  Did you do things or talk about things that were un-
    usual?

A:  Yes. My mother had died 1 year ago, and I phoned a
    friend something to the effect that she might think

that I didn't care much for my mother, and that
I didn't feel very badly about her. My mother was
very dear to me but when she died, I didn't wear
black and I didn't mourn. I seemed to feel that she
thought I didn't care about my mother's going.

**Q:** Was there anything unusual in the way you talked or
moved that made them think of a mental disease?

**A:** I didn't sleep for 1 week during that time. We had
several doctors. My mind was quite alert, possibly
too alert. My ears have always been alert, possibly,
too, a little too alert.[1]

**Q:** Didn't you think your husband would look on this
whole episode as quite a pointless thing?

**A:** I did, no I didn't at the time, but I have thought so
later.

**Q:** At the time, didn't it look like a rather foolish thing
to do?

**A:** At the time, it seemed to go out of my thoughts. I've
learned enough about hypnotism to know that one is
soothed by music and gotten into a sort of vacuum state.

**Q:** Did you feel you were under a hypnotic influence?

**A:** I felt I was being led at the time, but I don't know
whether I have wondered about it. I associated it
with the fact that there were men in the hotel lobby.

**Q:** What hotel lobby?

**A:** Where the party was to be.

**Q:** What were these men doing to you?

**A:** I don't know whether any of these men were working
with the idea that they would get it back at the in-
structors that were helping.

---

[1] *Note.* (Dictated by Dr. Woods) The patient drove around Kirksville to pass
the time until her social engagement was to begin. She drove outside the
town and picked up a hitch-hiker who announced that he wanted to go to
Des Moines. She offered to take him to the next town, and she felt that he
was saying to her that he might as well go with the patient beyond Des
Moines but did not actually say so. On reaching Des Moines, she went to the
home of a former acquaintance where she tried to telephone her husband
and explain her absence. Apparently, she had no purpose in mind when
going to Des Moines at that time.

Q: Why should you have gone to Des Moines?

A: You see, my husband and the board had divided the insurance. They might think that because I had talked things over with Mr. F. that it would have some influence on him.

Q: Why should you go to Des Moines instead of to the party?

A: It would be noticed that I would not be at the party. Most of the people would notice it and would think it an unusual thing I hadn't phoned that I was coming. They would wonder where I was and probably call Mr. F. in attempting to find out.

Q: What did all this have to do with the insurance?

A: They might want to make it unpleasant for Mr. F. by making me the type of person who was irresponsible. That would make him unhappy and might make trouble for him in his position.

Q: Did you want to make trouble for him?

A: No, but they did.

Q: Did this solution occur to you just now?

A: I think not. It came when I thought of those men. I had been to this hotel many times before to parties and I have never seen a crowd of men. At the time, I did not think of it as a hypnotic influence.

Q: Thank you very much, Mrs. F.

**Dr. Miller:** At the age of 32 we know that there had been no previous indication of a change in personality. The attacks have come on in regular cycles with the psychomotor activity tending to play a minor role. I think this is typical of the repeated manic depressive psychosis. The content seems to assume more importance as the psychomotor activity seems to drop out. I think we can understand that the manic patient with repeated attacks is depending more and more on rationalizing his behavior and the paranoid-like tendencies seem to come out as the disease becomes more prominent. I would feel that we are dealing with chronic manic depressive psychosis. I don't think the content is at all schizophrenic in

its makeup. It is the careless, superficial type of associations that one sees in mild mania without much
critical analysis of it.

**Dr. Gottlieb:**   I agree with Dr. Miller. It seems to be a
case of chronic mania. Interestingly, the lack of psychomotor activity is a rather poor prognostic sign
which is frequently seen associated with these cases.
I was interested in her formulations; particularly, the
logic as she demonstrated it is based almost entirely
on her feelings. She initiates every remark with
"I feel this" or "I feel that" and elaborates in a ra-
tional way on that basis, attempting to explain how
it could possibly have come about. The affect, although faulty and careless, does not show the schizophrenic deviations that one expects to see. The
associations do not appear to be schizophrenic. The
affect is certainly warm.[2]

## ▌ JMM

A 35-year-old, single, white woman was admitted April
1935. According to her physician, she had been depressed
and gloomy but had experienced active streaks and acted
in a childish, silly way for 3 weeks. When seen in the outpatient clinic on April 18, she was overactive, talkative, bel-
ligerent, uncooperative, sarcastic, and strenuously resisted
being taken to the ward. About 4 weeks before admission,
she seemed discouraged and very irritable. She was intru-
sive and interrupted other people. She had had some teeth
pulled and retained a mouth full of blood. When she returned home, she spit it into a fishbowl. She was hospitalized at another hospital a week prior to admission to the
University of Iowa and, during that time, was bored, not

---

[2] *Note.*   Doctors Lobb, Gottlieb, Miller, and Woods considered the patient's
condition as manic-depressive psychosis, manic. The other physicians
preferred undiagnosed psychosis. They recommended the patient be
discharged to the family, but the recommendation was not followed.
Instead, she was sent to another hospital.

very irritable, and did not seem either depressed or overactive, but she did talk in a superficial rambling and somewhat silly way.

Her past medical illness was significant in that, 5 years prior, she had experienced an illness similar to the present and was in a sanitarium for several months.

Her family history was positive. Her father had a period of melancholia, was discouraged, and stayed in bed a great deal. Her mother was in the state hospital at one time and was considered quite unstable. One brother was hospitalized in the state hospital for excessive alcoholism, and another was hospitalized in a psychiatric hospital and given a diagnosis of paranoid schizophrenia. He left home one night and was found dead the next morning lying face down in a shallow creek, presumably a suicide.

## April 18, 1935

Q:  How do you feel?
A:  Very well, thank you.
Q:  Are you sick?
A:  No.
Q:  Why are you in the hospital?
A:  For a rest.
Q:  Why do you need a rest?
A:  I don't need one.
Q:  Have you been working?
A:  Yes. I still am.
Q:  You are not working now, are you?
A:  I am still on the payroll.
Q:  You are not working right now, are you?
A:  Yes I am.
Q:  Why did you go to Mercy Hospital?
A:  Doctors' orders.
Q:  Why should he order it?
A:  You can't prove it by me.
Q:  I wonder why?
A:  The government is interested in professional people.
Q:  What has that got to do with it?
A:  That is the kind of work I have been in.

**Q:** What has that got to do with your being here?

**A:** Not a thing. I don't belong here.

**Q:** Did you get along all right down stairs?

**A:** I got into an argument.

**Q:** Why?

**A:** I have been educated. I was grabbed by two doctors.

**Q:** Why did they do that?

**A:** I was waiting to go back in the car.

**Q:** Has there been any change in your behavior recently?

**A:** I received good care.

**Q:** Have you felt any different lately?

**A:** I have been in the hospital before.

**Q:** Is there anything wrong with your mind?

**A:** No.

**Q:** Is your behavior the same as a year ago?

**A:** Yes.

**Q:** Have you ever had any nervous spells?

**A:** No. I am getting over it now. Everyone has a nervous system, don't they?

**Q:** Why did they send you here?

**A:** Yes, why should they? It was against my will.[3]

On May 2, she became excited, tried to get out of the ward, and refused to answer questions except for "goddamn yes" and "goddamn no." She made a remark that she would "like to light out of here and run like hell."

She did not improve and, on May 11, was transferred to a state hospital. At that time, her stream of talk was continuously pressured, and she was resentful about her hospitalization. During the whole time she was in the hospital, her mood was labile, generally elevated, and there were periods of manic excitement and silly conduct. On May 4, it was impossible to interview her because she would become excited, throw shoes around the room, and put her head under the water as if trying to drown herself. By September 1935, the state hospital reported back that she was still not sufficiently improved to justify a return home and

---

[3] *Note.* Dr. Malamud expressed the opinion that this was a mood disorder.

that she was still silly and uncontrollable, lacking judgment and insight. By the end of January 1936, it was felt that she had improved enough to get along outside of the hospital, and, by March 1936, she was released.

## ▎RUM

A 16-year-old schoolboy was brought to the hospital September 18, 1936, by his mother and two neighbors. He was shackled hand and foot. For the past week, he had been overtalkative and overactive. His first unusual behavior had been noted by his mother during the past summer when he began reading for long periods. In early September, he became talkative, too active, loud, boastful, and argumentative. Five days prior to admission, he had awakened one morning crying and told his mother that he "would have to go to Washington to tell the President to stop the war with Spain, and if necessary I will get ready and go to Spain myself in order to stop the war." He began talking very loudly about "war, school, the Pope, and Ethiopia."

He states that before admission he was very worried by many things, especially by his schoolwork.

### October 1, 1936

Q:  Why do you rhyme so much?
A:  I don't know why.
Q:  What did you mean by don't cross my eyes? Why are you so startled at noises?
A:  Because I'm a nervous wreck.
Q:  Why were you so concerned about the war in Spain?
A:  Because the rebels are Catholics like myself and I want them to win.

During the interview, the patient was startled by a lawn mower tractor passing the window. "That reminds me of a picture with Joe E. Brown. He pulled a house with an earthworm tractor; the people in it thought an earthquake had occurred; that reminded me of Quaker Oats, quake, afraid. That is why I was startled. I called Father Goretzsky 'Foxey' because his initials are FX." The physician noted that the patient talked off the subject at hand, rambled through his associations, kept eyes shut part of time, and rhymed freely and frequently.[4] His speech showed a good deal of pressure. That day he was tearful for the first time but only on references to home. This mood was probably copied from another patient who was tearful over going home and whom the patient was consoling just prior to the interview and to whom he makes references.

## October 7, 1936 (Progress Note)

The patient continues in a moderately active state. Placed in single room for brief periods because he jumps on beds. Last night voided and defecated in bed. In the morning spoke about it quite freely but could give only a number of obviously wrong reasons.

Today he said "I should keep quiet when I start to talk because what I say doesn't make sense. And I know I'm talking foolish. I do it all because I'm nervous."

During all the interviews he smiles quite freely and seems at ease. His movements are graceful, and his manner is bird-like and pert. He is always willing to talk, converses quietly, but, if left alone, he rambles around in his speech, rhymes, puns, and makes many apparently irrelevant remarks. He is greatly influenced by ward activities and especially the other patients. A surprising amount of his content is derived from the remarks of the other patients. He incorporates their talk and actions into his own, and at times it is difficult to differentiate between the content derived from himself and that from the other patients. "They said I am Will Rogers because I tried to be funny . . . Ego means you go before I go . . . I'd rather die for the church than for my country . . . I use Davis' (a patient) method and yell out the window for help . . . I crawled under the bed to show I'm meek."

---

[4] *Note.* Rhyme: Home sweet home, all roads lead to Rome, and men make poems.

## Staff Meeting: November 24, 1936

Q:  Good morning.

A:  Good morning.

Q:  How do you feel this morning?

A:  Just fine.

Q:  Are you quite happy?

A:  Yes, sir.

Q:  How much do you remember of what happened when you first came into the hospital?

A:  About three-fourths of the things.

Q:  Tell me some of the things you remember.

A:  I wanted to go home and ran around the room.

Q:  What else did you do?

A:  I broke the thermometer.

Q:  Why did you do that?

A:  I don't know.

Q:  You were talking about wanting to go to Spain. What was that about? What would you do in Spain?

A:  I'd fight.

Q:  Fight for what? Which side would you take?

A:  That's rather complicated.

Q:  There are two sides there. Which side would you take?

A:  The rebels are in one gang and . . .

Q:  You are not quite sure about it?

A:  No.

Q:  You do not know which of the two sides you would take if you were to go there but you would fight anyway.

A:  That's about it.

Q:  Do you still want to go to Spain?

A:  No.

Q:  Do you want to stay here now?

A:  Sure.

Q:  Do you feel quite as well now as you ever did in your life? Are you quite clear about things?

A:  Yes.

Q:  Do you think you are ready to go back to school?

A:  I am hoping I can.

**Q:**   What do you think happened? What was wrong with you?

**A:**   I had a nervous breakdown.

**Q:**   Did you ever have a nervous breakdown before?

**A:**   No, I didn't.

**Q:**   Has anybody you know ever had a nervous breakdown?

**A:**   No.

**Q:**   All right, Thanks for coming in.

**Dr. Malamud:**   Do you get the impression from talking to his people that this is his usual, normal self?

**Dr. Rodis:**   He is not quite back to normal. I asked the mother expressly about that.

**Dr. Malamud:**   Are the slight mannerisms and sheepish grin things he has had before?

**Dr. Rodis:**   The mother spoke especially about the fact that he has not been quite active enough in speech. He was quite embarrassed in here this morning.

**Dr. Malamud:**   Do we accept the diagnosis of manic-depressive, manic? (All accept diagnosis.) Do you think we ought to parole him and advise his people that he had better not go to school for the rest of the semester? (All agree to recommendation.) Whether he ought to go to school the second semester will depend on his condition when he returns from parole.

On November 27, the patient was paroled to his mother to return in 6 weeks for a check-up.

He seemed to do well. An interval history on January 9 showed that he was exhibiting no unusual ideas and functioning reasonably at home. He was admitted for a short period of observation between January 9 and January 14 and was discharged on January 14.

## January 14, 1937

**Q:**   Come in, R. Were you glad to come back to us?

**A:**   Sure.

**Q:**   Is it easier living here than at home?

**A:**   I don't know.

**Q:** Maybe we don't make you work so hard?

**A:** No.

**Q:** How much do you remember about when you were sick?

**A:** Some of it I forget.

**Q:** You were pretty sick for a while, weren't you?

**A:** Yes, I was.

**Q:** What do you remember about it?

**A:** I wouldn't eat.

**Q:** What made you do that way?

**A:** I don't know.

**Q:** Do you remember how you were when you first came here, what sort of things you were doing?

**A:** Things I shouldn't have.

**Q:** What kind of things were they?

**A:** I tried to get away.

**Q:** Did you cause any trouble?

**A:** Yes, I did.

**Q:** How was that?

**A:** I almost kicked the typewriter or something.

**Q:** What made you do that?

**A:** I don't know.

**Q:** Do you often kick typewriters?

**A:** No, I don't.

**Q:** Do you remember how you felt at that time that made you want to kick a typewriter?

**A:** No.

**Q:** Were you mad?

**A:** I might have been.

**Q:** Do you remember what made you mad?

**A:** Uh-huh.

**Q:** Maybe you were afraid of something. Did it seem to you that people were trying to do something to you?

**A:** I don't think they were.

**Q:** Do you remember any of the things you talked about then?

**A:** A few.

**Q:** What kind of things do you remember?

**A:** About Spain and the war.

**Q:** Had you been particularly interested in Spain?

**A:** Yes, I was.

**Q:** Were the people in Spain going to do something to you?

**A:** No.

**Q:** Then as you began to get better and felt more like yourself, do you remember things more clearly?

**A:** Quite a bit.

**Q:** What do you remember when you first began to be like yourself?

**A:** I remember talking to Dr. Rodis.

**Q:** Do you remember one morning getting up and feeling quite differently from the way you felt the day before? Did it change suddenly?

**A:** I don't think it did.

**Q:** There was a change, wasn't there?

**A:** Yes.

**Q:** Do you remember how you were sleeping then?

**A:** I didn't sleep very well.

**Q:** Are you sleeping all right now?

**A:** Better.

**Q:** Do you remember when that change came? Did it come gradually too?

**A:** Yes.

**Q:** About reading things, you can read things easily now. Could you when you were sick?

**A:** No, I couldn't.

**Q:** How much do you remember about the way you felt when this thing started? Do you remember when it started?

**A:** About Labor Day.

**Q:** The day before Labor Day you felt like your ordinary self?

**A:** Yes.

**Q:** And on Labor Day you felt different?

**A:** Yes, I did.

**Q:** Do you remember how you felt?

**A:** Well, I got poison ivy on me and that was cured but after that, I don't remember much.

**Q:** Then on Labor Day what else did you do that was unusual to you?

**A:** I went to a carnival and boxed.

**Q:** Did you feel different than your ordinary self?

**A:** I might have.

**Q:** Did you box in the same way you would have if you had not been sick?

**A:** I never had boxed much.

**Q:** Were you much excited when boxing? Did you do anything unusual?

**A:** I don't think I did.

**Q:** What happened on Labor Day that makes you fix that as the day it began?

**A:** I slept in school, was sort of sleepy.

**Q:** Now you want to go back and go to school?

**A:** Yes, I do.

**Q:** Do you feel like studying again?

**A:** Sure.

In February 1937, his mother indicated that he was doing satisfactorily. In September 1937, she reported that he was working and satisfied. When he returned for a follow-up visit, he was smiling, composed, and seemed ordinary. He was actually followed to November 1937, and there was no recurrence of his illness. He was leading his class academically, took part in athletics, and was well liked.

---

## The Schizophrenic Patients

### ▌ JLS

JLS was a 38-year-old, unmarried man. Seven and one-half years before his admission on December 11, 1935, he had quit his job as a telegraph operator and stayed home caring for his mother. About 1½ years prior to that admission, he had delusional ideas that the house was on fire and that the walls of the house were caving in, and he made a nuisance of himself by calling the fire department often. At examination, he was very vague and circumstantial, asking frequent, repetitious questions. He minimized his difficulties but admitted that he had a fear of fires, had been sleepless, and had worried about his mother. He stated that in 1928 he began to hear voices that would tell him to hurry; these voices also called him vulgar names and carried sexual connotations. He heard the voices of neighborhood girls that commanded him to carry out household duties. His emotional response seemed less than what would be expected considering the content of the thoughts. He was discharged January 12, 1936, to his home. His stay in the hospital was characterized by quietness, lack of communication, lack of initiative, and general dullness with delusions and hallucinations, which, for the most part, he later denied.

## January 8, 1936

**Q:**   Come in Mr. S.
**A:**   Hello.
**Q:**   What do you work at?
**A:**   I was a telegraph operator when I worked.
**Q:**   How long ago?
**A:**   Oh, I haven't worked for about 8 or 10 years.
**Q:**   Would you like to work?
**A:**   I liked it pretty well.
**Q:**   What made you give it up.
**A:**   After I got sick, I couldn't work very much.
**Q:**   Were you sick?
**A:**   Yes.
**Q:**   What was the matter?
**A:**   Flu, I guess.
**Q:**   And did that last long?
**A:**   Oh, about 2 weeks.
**Q:**   Then after you got well, did you want to go back?
**A:**   I went back after that. I worked for 3 years after that, and then I got sick again.
**Q:**   And then did you give it up completely?
**A:**   Almost.

**Q:** After your sickness was over, did you try to get back?

**A:** My mother got sick, and I didn't try to get back.

**Q:** How long have you been taking care of your mother?

**A:** Six years.

**Q:** Did you ever wish to get back into the work?

**A:** Oh yes.

**Q:** Why didn't you try to get back?

**A:** Oh, I don't know. I never tried very hard, I guess.

**Q:** Are you without much ambition?

**A:** No, I like to work.

**Q:** Why was it that you didn't make some effort to get back to work?

**A:** I lost my seniority and I couldn't get back in very well.

**Q:** Yes. Is there anything that is troubling you now?

**A:** No, doctor.

**Q:** Everything going nicely now?

**A:** Yes.

**Q:** Is your brother taking care of you?

**A:** Yes.

**Q:** Doesn't it ever trouble you that you are living off your brother now?

**A:** Yes.

**Q:** Then why is it that you do it? Wouldn't your friends admire you much more if you went out and got a job?

**A:** Yes.

**Q:** Do you care for girls?

**A:** Some.

**Q:** Ever think of getting married?

**A:** Not very much.

**Q:** Wouldn't it be better to get married and have your own family?

**A:** I suppose so. There is no hurry in it.

**Q:** How old are you?

**A:** 38.

**Q:** It is getting the time to do it if you are ever going to do it. What do you think of girls? Do you enjoy them?

**A:** Yes.

**Q:** Do you get along nicely with them?

A: Yes.

Q: Have you ever had a good girl friend?

A: Yes, I have.

Q: Do you like to go with girls? Have you ever taken one to a movie?

A: I used to when I was working. After I stopped, I didn't care much for it.

Q: Do girls like you?

A: I don't know.

Q: Do they ever show that they are interested in you?

A: I guess so.

Q: Do you go to church?

A: Yes, sir.

Q: What church?

A: Catholic church. I haven't gone for a long time.

Q: Does it help you?

A: Yes.

Q: How long ago did you go last?

A: Just before I came down here I went to the priest and confessed.

Q: Do you believe in spirits?

A: No.

Q: What do you think about telepathy? Are people able to talk to you from a distance?

A: I don't know about that.

Q: Was there a time that people across the way talked to you and told you things?

A: I don't know.

Q: Have you ever had experiences of that sort that seemed a little peculiar?

A: I think I did.

Q: We are interested in that sort of thing and would like to hear about it. Tell us about it.

A: I guess it was more like imagination.

Q: And what did it feel like?

A: Oh (pause), I used to have a hard time to get up in the morning, and they knew that I didn't like to get up, and there is sort of a lot of imagination.

Q: And what did they do?

A: They would yell it is time to get up now.

Q: Did it seem to be voices of particular people that you knew?

A: I think they did.

Q: Was it women's voices?

A: Yes.

Q: Friends of yours?

A: Maybe it was.

Q: What effect did it have on you? Did it frighten you?

A: No.

Q: How long ago was it?

A: A little time before I came down here.

Q: Since you have been in the hospital, have you heard things of that sort?

A: No.

Q: How do people around you think about you? Are they nice to you and are they kind to you?

A: Yes.

Q: Is there anybody doing things against you?

A: No.

Q: Do you plan to go back home and continue living the same way?

A: I would like to go back to work.

Q: And will you try to go back to work?

A: Yes. I don't know how it will go because I lost my seniority.

Q: After you go home, will there still be danger of walls falling down and things happening?

A: I don't think so.

Q: Why won't there be?

A: It was all brought on by excessive smoking.

Q: Were you taking medicine then?

A: Yes.

Q: What was the medication?

A: I don't know the name, something for my nerves.

Q: How long were you taking it?

A: A couple of weeks.

Q: And was it only then that the house seemed to be in danger.

A: About that time.

Q: Alright, that will be enough this morning.

The patient's maternal grandfather had a brother who was said to have been strange, but there was no other history of nervous illness in the family.

A letter on April 26, 1938, indicated he was still about the same—still deluded and hallucinating, and he said that everyone had syphilis. He often stayed in bed until noon and answered questions with only a "yup" or a "nope." In July 1944, a letter from the state hospital arrived stating he had a loosely connected paranoid trend of thought, and he believed that he was Christ returned to earth for the second time.

# ▌ JKS

A 34-year-old unmarried woman had been expressing ideas of reference and persecution. She said that her nervousness was caused by persecution by a number of people who had used her since she was born for the purpose of making motion pictures. They had cameras concealed in electric lights and in the walls, and they watched her every time she went anywhere and then released her pictures under somebody else's name instead of hers. Thus, she had played as Ruby Keeler in *42nd Street,* and she was the star in pictures that were released under the name of Joan Crawford, Jean Harlow, and others. The directors of these motion pictures kept on pestering her by continually talking to her, giving her "lines" to which she was forced to respond.

She was admitted in October 16, 1934. Her difficulties had started insidiously. The first abnormality was noticed in June 1933 when she declared to her mother that the mother was not her mother but that she, the patient, was an adopted child and that possibly she had several mothers. Then she remarked that people were not real to her, and she sat for hours absorbed in her own thoughts, often giggling to herself. Though she was bright and trained as a teacher, she had not done anything for the 2 years prior to admission. She was in the hospital for less than a month. During that time, she remarked that she was the victim of an organization that was placing photographic apparatuses into "lightholes" in order to obtain moving pictures of her. She said that things had not been natural to her for most of her life, and she told a symbolic story of two children who went into the woods and were varnished by a witch so that they were like two dolls and couldn't move. She felt that she was varnished that way and had to be salvaged by the magic word of her mother, just as the children were by their mother. Then she said it is not she who was varnished, but the rest of the world, and that things did not look natural.

Her mood was sometimes playful, mostly contented, sometimes apathetic. Prior to her discharge on November 9, the following interview was performed:

Q: I see they have taken your intelligence quotient this morning.

A: Yes.

Q: Did you like it?

A: No.

Q: You came out very nicely.

A: Thanks.

Q: Do you feel that you have been very different from other people in your earlier life?

A: I think that my early life has been very different, but I don't think I have been especially different.

Q: In what way was your life different?

A: I couldn't tell you that in a million years.

Q: Was your life different from that of your brothers and sisters?

A: I don't know if I have any brothers and sisters.

Q: Are there people you have called brothers and sisters?

A: Brothers.

Q: Was your early life very different from that of your brothers?

A: No, not very much different.

Q: Did you feel all along that your capacity and ambi-

tions made you a little different from ordinary
people?

**A:** No I haven't felt that.

**Q:** When did you first begin to feel that.

**A:** You said ambition and capacities—well they are two
different things. I felt that my capacity was different
only very recently. Regarding my ambition, I don't
know. I always thought I was ambitious in some
respects.

**Q:** What is your greatest ambition now?

**A:** To get out.

**Q:** And when you get out and establish yourself in the
world, what do you want to become?

**A:** Myself.

**Q:** I am interested in knowing just what kind of a self
you can become?

**A:** That would be a guess. I don't know.

**Q:** In what kind of life would you shine most?

**A:** I don't want to shine.

**Q:** In what kind of life would you succeed best?

**A:** Just ordinary, every day life.

**Q:** Has this ability that you have to pose as a movie
actress been easily acquired?

**A:** No.

**Q:** Is it just a matter of capacity or have you thought of
it and trained yourself?

**A:** I have not thought and trained myself, of that I am
sure.

**Q:** When did you think it was first discovered?

**A:** By myself or others?

**Q:** By yourself.

**A:** I didn't know that I had any ability until just recently.

**Q:** When you discovered that you had this ability, how
did you come to realize it?

**A:** Suggestions.

**Q:** Who suggested it?

**A:** Several people.

**Q:** Your friends thought and told you you had ability?

**A:** They didn't tell me.

Q:   How was it suggested?

A:   Oh by just rather vague hints now and then.

Q:   Are there cameras being focused on you now?

A:   I suppose so.

Q:   How can you discern that?

A:   As I said several times, I am becoming very tense.

Q:   Do you feel tense now.

A:   Yes, I do.

Q:   Do you feel sure that there are cameras being focused on you now although we can't hear them or see them?

A:   I am not sure of anything.

Q:   So when you say they are being used, you are not sure about it?

A:   I don't really mean that.

Q:   Just what is it you mean?

A:   In this world you are not definitely sure of anything, are you?

Q:   How did you get that idea?

A:   I am sure I don't know.

Q:   Do you realize that that sort of statement has made your friends very uneasy about you? They feel that something is wrong with your mind.

A:   Can it be possible that they are uneasy about me?

Q:   Here you are an intelligent girl, educated, trained for teaching and yet you sit before us and tell us that moving picture machines are being used to photograph you right at this moment when not one of us see any reason to think that that is true. Isn't that important?

A:   Not to me it isn't.

Q:   Do you realize that when your friends become uneasy about such things, if they think your mind is diseased, they will take you to a hospital for the insane?

A:   In the first place, do I have any friends and who are they? In the second place, are you right or am I or are you just talking to me? In the third place, I have a definite idea that I am not going to an insane asylum.

**Q:** If we should find that I happen to be right and you are wrong and someone will come in a day or two and take you to a state hospital, would that be a serious thing?

**A:** Very serious.

**Q:** What would you do about it?

**A:** I would do my best about it.

**Q:** I am anxious to advise you about it. What could you do under the circumstances?

**A:** I would have to know if it were a real state hospital or not, and then that would determine my course of action.

**Q:** Wouldn't it be advisable for you to show us that there is real reason for these beliefs so that we can respect them?

**A:** I think you think I am all right. It is obvious that I am all right. The thing for you to do is to prove you are all right.

**Q:** Five or 6 years ago, what did you think of the movie world?

**A:** I didn't think much of it.

**Q:** Did it interest you much?

**A:** Not any more than usual.

**Q:** Do you always approve of the type of shows put out?

**A:** Not always.

**Q:** Some are indecent?

**A:** Yes.

**Q:** Have these people actually intruded in your room?

**A:** I have never held the camera in my hands, but I feel sure that they have taken advantage of me.

**Q:** You mean in postures and dress that made you ashamed?

**A:** Yes.

**Q:** You saw the production?

**A:** Yes.

**Q:** You could recognize yourself?

**A:** Yes, after I came to.

**Q:** Came to from what?

**A:** I have to explain that. When I found out I was working for the movies, there were different actors who were doubled for me.

**Q:** When you say actors doubled for you, what do you mean?

**A:** I don't know.

**Q:** Did they photograph others and represent it as you?

**A:** I suppose. I don't know what they did and I don't care.

**Q:** If they can arrange it so that cameras are present in the room, would it be difficult to prevent it?

**A:** Very.

**Q:** They must be intangible cameras that cannot be seen. Is that possible?

**A:** No, I think they are tangible to you.

**Q:** Where, for instance, in this room could they be?

**A:** In the lights—I don't know.

**Q:** If when you were teaching school one of your students had said that an electric light might contain a camera, what would you have said to the child?

**A:** I don't know. I believe everything.

**Q:** If you were teaching today and some child said it, what would you tell the child?

**A:** I would say it is possible.

**Dr. W. Woods:** I think we are dealing with schizophrenia of the paranoid type. This patient reminds me somewhat of the M case. She shows retention of a great deal of paranoid affect, and, yet, the particular type of associations going with it is very much disturbed. I can very well imagine she is a very difficult case to deal with. If a proper amount of supervision could be given outside, I think she could be cared for at home.

**Dr. Woods:** When you spoke about her retaining a great deal of paranoid affect, did you mean she seemed to be capable of flashes of irritation?

**Dr. W. Woods:** Yes.

**Dr. Woods:** Were you impressed with anything particular connected with the psychogenic field?

**Dr. Malamud:** There is nothing that I can consider as a possibility. Undoubtedly, there was some kind of

experience that made her reach out for these imagi-
nations, but I don't see anything that could be taken
as a possible psychogenic cause. I think too that this
is schizophrenia of the paranoid type. I don't see
very much proper affect and although we do see a
certain kind of flash, it is a lukewarm type. As to the
disposition, I suppose she could be tried outside, but
I feel her people would have to be warned. Also, it
seems to me that if there is any hope for improvement, the fact that she would be allowed to go home
and get back to her old thoughts might interfere
with her getting over it.

**Dr. Woods:**   There was nothing we could get at in her
past life that indicated an interest in her own figure
or gracefulness. She had not gone in for physical development?

**Dr. Lindemann:**   No, there was nothing of that type.

**Dr. Woods:**   It does look as though she must have
thought over and dreamed over this matter of
appearing as a movie actress. There were no love
affairs?

**Dr. Lindemann:**   She went with a young man for some-
time, but there was never any emotional intensity.

**Dr. Woods:**   The fault in her personality has been obvious from the first as she has constantly flitted from
one position to another, feeling that she was not being given a fair chance. As to the disposition, I feel
that the more protected life of a state hospital, the
routine, and freedom from competition and disturbance that she would not have at home might be
beneficial to her.

**Dr. Malamud:**   The brother was very much interested in
her and it is quite possible that he may want to take
her out even though we feel that state hospitalization is advisable.

The patient's diagnosis was schizophrenia, paranoid type,
and she was recommended to a state hospital but allowed
to go home if relatives insisted. Her relatives took her

home. In March 1935, the patient's brother reported that she had experienced three periods when she thought everybody was against her and was particularly antagonistic toward her mother. She showed no interest in music, which had formerly been her vocation, but had learned to help her mother around the house. She had given up her ideas that she was a movie star and that people were photographing her. She did some driving but showed no interest in outside activities. In January 1936, she no longer spoke of being a motion picture star and never spoke of any peculiar happenings. She seemed content to stay home and made no effort to go out socially. She seemed childlike and dependent. In February 1937, her mother wrote and noted that she did some driving and some household shopping. The patient said she was anxious to get away for a vacation with someone who would "help her separate the real from the unreal." In September 1937, her brother reported that she had the idea that she now had a large number of children who were being kept from her by her mother. By July 1938, the patient's brother thought that her condition was greatly improved, but she was not completely cured. The time between her episodes of suspiciousness was longer, but occasionally she expressed delusions. She was interviewed at home in April 1938, and, although she seemed neat in appearance, the doctor said she still believed that she was a movie star. She was considered unimproved. Her family history was negative for mental disease.

## ▌ JDS

A 24-year-old male had been ill for about 6 months prior to admission. He had peculiar ideas; for example, he thought that he had to marry someone, that he had ear trouble, and that there was something wrong with his head. He felt he wasn't on a par with other people, cried, and had become relatively asocial, spending most of his time at home. He had threatened suicide. On one occasion, he jumped out of bed and ran around the room. He broke the chairs over his head, stating that there was a pressure there that he had to break. He thought that everybody was critical of him. He was admitted May 18, 1938, and discharged June 11. On May 20, a progress note was written that contained some verbatim material from an interview.

## Progress Note: May 20, 1938

The patient was admitted to the hospital only after two attendants had gone to the automobile and forcefully brought him to the ward. During the physical examination, he was suspicious, frequently said "now, is that necessary?" but was not uncooperative. Since admission, his behavior has been somewhat better. He refused to eat supper until he was threatened with tube feeding and since then has eaten well.

Q:  Why are you here?

A:  I don't know, but last night there were like moving pictures with music all around in my room for inebriates.

Q:  What was the story of the movie?

A:  Really, I don't know that. There were things that reminded me of people back home. It was like an inspiration. Really there was a man who talked about his movie and then the inspiration that I was part of the movie came to me. It seemed as if the food I was taking here held me down.

Q:  Have you had any funny feelings?

A:  I did last night. When I walked across the room it seemed as if the music was following me.

Q:  Where did the music seem to come from?

A:  Not recorded music but from a band, probably from the radio.

Q:  Anything else?

A:  Yes, sounds of an engine—a stream line train and I think I heard a fog horn once.

Q:  Where would a fog horn be around here?

A:  Possibly from the river.

Q:  Any voices?

A:  I can't say that I did, not directly any way.

Q: Indirectly?

A: Dr. B and the woman who is supposed to be his wife gave me some tip offs that made me feel pretty good. This supposed Mrs. B is acting for my girlfriend and he is my double. She comes at night when I am asleep.

Q: Have you been thinking about your girlfriend a lot?

A: (No answer given)

## Progress Note: May 27, 1938

The patient's behavior has remained about the same. He eats and sleeps fairly well. He is at times quite loud and aggressive, but there have been no definite outbreaks. He is quite insulting at times, especially to certain nurses and attendants, and is always very suspicious. On interviews, he is querulous and suspicious but gives a fairly good story. He dates the onset of his present illness to the age of 17 at which time a farm hand with whom he was sleeping had sexual relations with him intra-ano. Though he did not realize what was happening because he was asleep, he feels that the shock to his nervous system has wrecked his life. He elaborates at length concerning the various peculiar things that are happening in the hospital, feeling that the local papers are full of things which refer to him and he feels that frequent reference is made to him over the radio. He persists in the idea that the reason for his hospital stay is that he is the hero of a movie which is being taken but he does not know what the movie is about.

## June 7, 1938

Q: What did you do yesterday to pass the time?

A: Well, I . . . read a little, took some exercise, ate my food.

Q: Do you like living here?

A: Well, I can't say as I do.

Q: What do you intend to do when you get out?

A: Depends on what shape I get out in.

**Q:** What shape will you get out in?

**A:** I hope to go out in good health at least.

**Q:** Aren't you in good health now?

**A:** I can't say that.

**Q:** What is the trouble now?

**A:** (Laughs) Well, I just feel like I'm all shrunk up.

**Q:** Where abouts? Your face looks natural.

**A:** It don't seem natural.

**Q:** Your arms and legs look about the right size.

**A:** But they don't feel that way.

**Q:** Tell me about it.

**A:** Well . . . it just feels like everything is pulled together, don't feel natural, out of shape (laughs).

**Q:** What shape do you suppose you are in?

**A:** Might be hypnotized.

**Q:** Does it make you look like something else than yourself?

**A:** Well, to a certain extent it does.

**Q:** Like what, for instance?

**A:** Probably through members of my family, maybe, or in different stages.

**Q:** You say you think you look as though you were hypnotized.

**A:** I can't say I look that way but can imagine that maybe I feel that way.

**Q:** Have you any idea who it is hypnotizing you?

**A:** I can't be sure of that.

**Q:** Why should they want to hypnotize you?

**A:** (Laughs) Well, that remains to be seen.

**Q:** Do you suppose there is someone who wants you to do certain things or think certain things?

**A:** Probably.

**Q:** What kind of things would that be?

**A:** Maybe is like things or . . .

**Q:** Is it just to change your general appearance or change your interest?

**A:** Probably actions maybe—actions maybe.

**Q:** Do you like this to go on? Are you glad it is going on?

**A:** Well, it is . . . I think it is going on quite a while.

Q: Are you glad it is going on? Is it going to do you good or might it hurt you?

A: Well, I can't be sure of that.

Q: When you speak of people hypnotizing you, do they ever seem to be putting thoughts into your mind or talking to you?

A: Probably.

Q: How far do they go in that?

A: Not very far, just to the impulse so you can just barely gather the thought or what they might be thinking or what they want you to think.

Q: Can you hear them talking to you?

A: I never hear any voices.

Q: Do they ever appear so you can see them?

A: Not exactly.

Q: Do you see them in your dreams?

A: Yes.

Q: Are they people you know?

A: Yes.

Q: It is only in your dreams they come to you?

A: In actual vision, yes.

Q: You mean while you are awake?

A: No, while I am asleep.

Q: Do they talk to you in your dreams?

A: No, I can't be sure they do.

Q: What sort of thoughts is it they put into your mind?

A: . . . Am I bound to talk? Am I under obligations to express myself?

Q: We would like you to talk so we can understand just what the whole thing is.

A: Well, how far? Shouldn't there be some stopping point?

Q: Well, you are friendly to us and we are friendly to you. Why should there be a stopping point? You mean these people are trying to make some very serious change in you?

A: I can't be sure of that.

Q: Is there something that is difficult to say, something you are ashamed of?

A: I can't say there is.

Q: In general, what sort of thing is it they are putting into your mind?

A: Well, it might be a change of opinion. It may be a difference in looks or might be a different environment. It is fairly complicated, in other words.

Q: What will you do about this? Will you go ahead and let them do things to you?

A: Well, I don't know what I will do.

Q: Are you religious?

A: Well, (laughs) I wouldn't say I am so religious.

Q: Do you suppose the spirits have anything to do with it, God or the angels?

A: I don't know.

Q: When these people influence you, are they doing it by way of spirits, or do the Masons or organizations of that sort or the Catholic church have anything to do with it?

A: I don't know but I belong to the Catholic church. If I remember right, they have powers to do certain things. I can't say that about other religions, I don't know.

Q: Are there people in this hospital joining in this?

A: There might be.

Q: Have you noticed anything peculiar going on?

A: Well, I can't be sure of it but I think maybe there is.

## Progress Note: June 8, 1938

The patient's behavior remains very much the same. He is at times resistive to care and has to be secluded for a while, but most of the time he is on the ward. He continually insists that there is something wrong with his left ear and that it should be opened. One night he was sure that his mother was outside the ward door as he heard her talking. Today he refused to eat and tonight it was necessary to tube feed him. While being packed for the feeding he said, "I am being crucified" but cooperated very nicely in swallowing the tube. He was discharged June 11.

## Post Interview: Staff Conference

**Dr. Woods:**   It is a question whether these very loosely connected ideas should be considered paranoid. It is pretty much the phantasmic form of schizophrenia. Often you see just a degree of loose phantasy in ordinary hebephrenia, and his whole makeup makes me incline a little toward that diagnosis. There is evidence of marked deterioration in his emotional reactions. I would not fuss with either diagnosis. The absence of clear-cut hallucinations makes one lean a little toward the paranoid type.

**Dr. Orr:**   The length of the illness, I think, would make one think of the paranoid form of schizophrenia.

**Dr. Woods:**   That is often the case, too, in hebephrenia.

**Dr. Render:**   I think I should prefer to call it the paranoid type.

**Dr. Buxton:**   I should prefer the diagnosis of hebephrenia.

**Dr. Miller:**   I would call it hebephrenia because it is so scattered and silly, without definite systematization to the delusions. Most paranoid schizophrenics are apt to be quite concerned about their persecution or the belief that they are involved in some grandiose system, that they have enemies or that their food is poisoned.

**Dr. Lobb:**   I think on the whole I would agree with Dr. Miller.

**Dr. Woods:**   The majority is in favor of hebephrenia. State hospitalization is necessary.

The patient's diagnosis was schizophrenia, hebephrenia, and he was recommended to a state hospital.

The family history was positive for mental disease. His father had experienced a nervous breakdown about 20 years earlier and had been hospitalized for about 6 months at a state hospital. He had some odd ideas but insisted that he always knew what he was doing. No other member of the family had any psychiatric problems.

In April 1939, the state hospital reported that the patient showed no improvement and that he was very delusional. His delusions were largely of a religious and paranoid nature. He compared himself with Christ and had the feeling he was being sent to the hospital to save the world. He was hallucinating, often irritable, sullen, and did not associate with other patients. He was paroled on March 8, 1939, from the state hospital but was no better; if anything, it was felt that he might be getting worse.

# ▌ LALS

A 21-year-old, single woman was admitted for increasing inefficiency, refusal to speak or associate with others, and hallucinatory experiences. These symptoms of illness had begun around 2 months prior to admission on July 27, 1936. The patient thought she could hear men discussing her as early as November of 1935, when she was riding to and from school in streetcars. This evolved, and by May she thought that friends and possibly relatives were directing her by mental telepathy. When seen in the hospital, she was aloof and showed a great deal of giggling, grimacing, and some posturing. Her speech was disconnected and interwoven with irrelevant details.

## Staff Rounds: July 31, 1936

Q: Where are you?
A: (Smiles—no reply)
Q: You smile as if you were happy.
A: (No reply)
Q: It takes you a long time to answer.
A: Yes (whispers)
Q: What makes you like to talk?
A: When there is a good reason for talking.
Q: And a good reason is not present now?
A: (No reply)
Q: Have you a good many friends?
A: (Smiles)

**Q:** What did the fortune teller tell you to do?

**A:** (Looks puzzled)

**Q:** Is it a good thing to do?

**A:** (No reply)

**Q:** How would you know what was good for you?

**A:** (Smiles)

**Q:** Do you not answer because you dislike talking about fortune tellers?

**A:** (Nods head "no")

**Q:** Is it because you are not cautious?

**A:** No.

**Q:** Do you notice that is different than you used to be?

**A:** Yes.

**Q:** Has something changed to make you feel differently toward people?

**A:** (Smiles)

**Q:** What do you want to make of yourself?

**A:** (Smiles) I don't know (whispers)

**Q:** Do words or thoughts come to you through windows?

**A:** Not now.

**Q:** When they did, were they pleasant things? Could you make out what they were talking about?

**A:** (Tears. No reply)

**Q:** Are you happy to be here? Do you want to stay here a long time?

**A:** (Tearful)

**Q:** What is this place? Do you know the name of it?

**A:** No.

**Q:** What is the name of the town?

**A:** Iowa City.

**Q:** What sort of place is it? Factory, shop, hotel, or what?

**A:** (Smiles) It's a sanitarium for mental cases.

**Q:** Is that your trouble?

**A:** Yes.

**Q:** Is your mind troubled?

**A:** Yes.

**Q:** How does your mind feel? How is it troubled? Does it feel different, good, happy, etc.?

A:  It is not unhappy but it is different.

Q:  Do you like it?

A:  (Smiles) No.

Q:  Would you like to go back to what you call normal,
    or do you want to stay this way?

A:  I would like to have my mind normal.

Q:  What makes you think it isn't behaving itself?

A:  (No reply)

Q:  Why do you talk in a whisper?

A:  It hurts my throat to talk.

Q:  Has it been sore for some time? Does it hurt to eat?

A:  No.

## Staff Meeting: September 10, 1936

Q:  Good morning, Miss S. How are you getting along?

A:  Beg pardon?

Q:  How do you feel this morning?

A:  I feel fair.

Q:  Not quite well, is that it? What seems to be the
    trouble?

A:  I am far from being well.

Q:  What seems to be the trouble? You say you are not
    feeling well. Is there something that is hurting you
    or worrying you? What makes you feel not quite well?

A:  Well, I'm nervous.

Q:  Tell me about it.

A:  My head aches.

Q:  What else?

A:  Well, my eyes blur and my complexion is broken out
    and I'm nervous.

Q:  You are nervous? What do you mean by that?

A:  Nervous—well, my body is nervous.

Q:  Your body is nervous. What do you mean by that?

A:  In different ways.

Q:  That doesn't tell me very much either. In what way?
    Give me some examples.

A:  Well, I have a nervousness in my stomach.

Q:  How does that express itself?

A: (No reply)

Q: Does the whole thing seem funny and not important to you?

A: Of course not.

Q: You are talking in this way, sort of laughing at it.

A: That is the nervousness.

Q: Tell me about your stomach. How does it seem nervous to you?

A: It seems to affect my stomach.

Q: What?

A: This nervousness.

Q: So this nervousness affects your stomach and your stomach is nervous. What does that mean?

A: It just does, it seems to.

Q: What does your stomach do that makes you think it is nervous?

A: (No reply)

Q: Do you vomit?

A: No.

Q: Do you have any pain in your stomach?

A: No.

Q: What is it you would say is wrong with your stomach?

A: I can't explain.

Q: Maybe there is nothing wrong with it?

A: Yes, there is.

Q: There is something wrong with it but you can't explain it?

A: I move my hands a lot.

Q: And what else? Are other parts of your body affected by it?

A: My feet.

Q: How do your feet show this nervousness.

A: They move.

Q: You are a little bit restless and fidgety?

A: Yes.

Q: How long has that been going on?

A: A long time.

Q: How long is a long time? All your life?

A: Yes.

**Q:** You have had this stomach nervousness all your life?

**A:** At times.

**Q:** But it has been getting worse recently?

**A:** (No reply)

**Q:** Why do you laugh when I ask these things? Do they seem funny to you?

**A:** Occasionally.

**Q:** What seems funny to you, the fact I am asking these questions or the fact that these things exist?

**A:** In some respects.

**Q:** Tell me, this nervousness has become definitely worse recently, hasn't it?

**A:** (No reply)

**Q:** Has it?

**A:** (No reply)

**Q:** Tell me, what would you say has happened recently to make things worse?

**A:** Well, nervous eating.

**Q:** You mean you have been eating in a way that has affected your health?

**A:** I don't know.

**Q:** What do you mean by nervous eating?

**A:** (No reply)

**Q:** Do you mean too fast, too slow, too much or too little?

**A:** Too much, I think.

**Q:** And you think because of that you have become a little nervous?

**A:** I don't think that is the cause of that.

**Q:** Tell me what was the question I asked in the beginning?

**A:** About food?

**Q:** I didn't ask you about food. Just before you told me about nervous eating, what was the question I asked you?

**A:** Whether I had been more nervous since I've been here.

**Q:** And then what did I ask you?

**A:** (No reply)

**Q:** I asked what had caused you to be more nervous and you said nervous eating.

**A:** (No reply)

**Q:** Tell me, has anything unusual been going on within the last 2 or 3 months?

**A:** Yes.

**Q:** What?

**A:** I can't explain it.

**Q:** Explain it as much as you can.

**A:** I have been hearing talking.

**Q:** What do you mean by that? Don't all of us hear when people talk?

**A:** Of course.

**Q:** What is the difference between your experiences and ours?

**A:** Mine seems to come in a different manner.

**Q:** By that you mean what?

**A:** I don't know.

**Q:** When people are in the room with you and they talk, you hear them. Is that it?

**A:** I don't know.

**Q:** When people are in the room with you and they talk, you hear them. Is that it?

**A:** What?

**Q:** When people in the room with you talk, you hear them?

**A:** Of course.

**Q:** Is there anything else, anything unusual about the situation?

**A:** No.

**Q:** There is nothing unusual about hearing people talk when they are with you?

**A:** No.

**Q:** Why mention the fact that you hear people talking?

**A:** It's in a different manner.

**Q:** You mean by that what?

**A:** I don't know exactly.

**Q:** Do you mean you have heard people talking even when they were not there?

A:  Yes.

Q:  Why didn't you say that when I asked you about something unusual?

A:  I think I did.

Q:  What did these people say?

A:  Different things.

Q:  Of course they would say different things. What did they talk about?

A:  Well, most of it doesn't make sense, occasionally it does.

Q:  What are some of the things they say that don't make sense?

A:  Well, I can't think of anything.

Q:  How do you know then it doesn't make sense?

A:  It didn't make sense to me.

Q:  What do they say? Do you recognize these people when you hear the voices?

A:  Not now, I did.

Q:  When you did recognize them, who were they?

A:  Ruth, my cousin.

Q:  Where was she at the time you heard her talking?

A:  I don't know.

Q:  She was not with you?

A:  Well, the talking sounded in a different way.

Q:  Let's get this clear. She was not with you at the time?

A:  No.

Q:  And you heard her talking?

A:  Yes.

Q:  Did she address you?

A:  No.

Q:  Did she talk about you?

A:  No, that is, I don't know some of it.

Q:  Some of it was about you?

A:  Some of it was addressed to a second person.

Q:  You mean she was talking to some other person?

A:  No, some of it was addressed—some of it was addressed to me. I don't know whether it was addressed to me.

Q:  What are some of the things she said?

A:  Well, it don't make any particular sense. I didn't hear any—It seemed she said "relax" continually.

Q:  You thought they meant you should relax?

A:  Yes.

Q:  Was it Ruth talking about relaxation or somebody else?

A:  It seemed to be her voice. I heard voices about three different ways. I mean they seemed—

Q:  The voices came in three different ways?

A:  Yes.

Q:  What were the three different ways? What do you mean?

A:  Some of it seemed to be people talking, actually talking. Some of it just seemed to be in my mind; I can't exactly explain it. Some of it seemed to be coming a different way besides.

Q:  Some of it was like people actually talking, like I am here now. Was it loud or a whisper?

A:  Most of it was not very loud.

Q:  Just ordinary talking?

A:  Yes.

Q:  And the other way was that these things seemed to be going through your mind but you couldn't hear them?

A:  Yes. This is, they are like sounds or like thoughts— not thoughts.

Q:  They are words and yet there is no sound to them?

A:  Well, some of it doesn't have sense and some does.

Q:  What is the third way like?

A:  Some of it seems to be real talking and some of it just seems to be in my mind. I am being made to think it is talk; I can't very well explain it.

Q:  You said there were three different ways; you have given only two.

A:  I mean hearing ordinary talking—well, I've tried to explain it.

Q:  You said some of it was like ordinary talking and some of it just seemed to be in your mind. What is the third way?

**A:** Some of it seems to be just in my mind and some of it seems to be actual talking in some other way.

**Q:** What is the third way?

**A:** Actual talking, some of it. That is—well, of course, if you actually hear people talking, you hear them talking and they are usually rather close to you. This other seems to be different. It seems to be actual— well, I can't explain it.

**Q:** What do you think about it? Do you think people actually are talking or is it your imagination?

**A:** I don't think it could be my imagination.

**Q:** People are actually talking to you?

**A:** It seems they are.

**Q:** Yet you don't see actual people; how can you hear their voices?

**A:** (No reply).

**Q:** Did you hear any last night?

**A:** Yes.

**Q:** Who was talking last night?

**A:** I don't know.

**Q:** Men or women?

**A:** I hear men's voices sometimes.

**Q:** Last night did you hear men's voices?

**A:** Yes.

**Q:** Where were you at the time you heard them?

**A:** Well, different places.

**Q:** Where were you at the time you heard them?

**A:** Well, at different times . . .

**Q:** Pick out some special time when you heard them, where were you at the time?

**A:** When I would be cleaning.

**Q:** Would there be other people with you?

**A:** No.

**Q:** Yet you could hear these people talking and it sounded like regular voices?

**A:** Yes.

**Q:** What did they say?

**A:** Well, I can't remember exactly.

**Q:** Can't you remember approximately? What was the

nature of the things they talked about? Did they say some bad things about you?

A: (No reply).

Q: What did they say about you?

A: You didn't . . .

Q: What did they say about you?

A: It didn't make sense.

Q: You don't remember at all what they said?

A: No.

Q: How do you know you heard it? Maybe you didn't hear it.

A: Yes, I did.

Q: Do you hear any now?

A: No.

Q: Did you hear any when you first came into the room?

A: No.

Q: When people talk to you, you know they are near. That is the normal way of hearing things.

A: Yes.

Q: When people are talking to you this way, do you hear voices coming in from somewhere else?

A: No.

Q: Do they sometimes break into a conversation?

A: No.

Q: Is it only when you are by yourself that you can hear them?

A: Yes.

Q: What makes you hear these voices when we can't hear them?

A: I don't know.

Q: You do have ideas about it, don't you?

A: No.

Q: You talked about the possibility of some person hypnotizing you?

A: Yes.

Q: So you did talk about it. Why should this person hypnotize you, what good would it do him?

A: I don't know.

**Q:** How does he do that? Does he go into your room and hypnotize you?

**A:** No.

**Q:** How does he do it?

**A:** I don't know.

**Q:** What is going to be the outcome of all this thing? Have you been thinking about it, trying to make plans?

**A:** I don't know; I can't make any plans?

**Q:** Would you like someone to help you get rid of these things or would you just as soon go on hearing them?

**A:** Of course—of course I want to get rid of them.

**Q:** All right, Miss S, thank you for coming in.

## Staff Meeting Following the Interview

**Dr. Malamud:** Dr. Gottlieb, tell me why does Dr. Lovell say this is schizophrenia?

**Dr. Gottlieb:** Because of the symptoms she has presented: In the first place, the affect is very considerably affected as one can see by her inappropriate reactions, the silly type of smiling that is continually breaking through which is not at all suitable to the thought content and which does not seem to have any particular meaning. Also, she has been withdrawn from others, has been listening to her hallucinatory experiences, and is considerably enwrapped with her inner experiences. In addition, reality has been changed for her.

**Dr. Malamud:** Is there a disturbance of reality in her concepts?

**Dr. Gottlieb:** Not necessarily in concepts but in her experiences. That is often allied with schizophrenia.

**Dr. Malamud:** If you were to use that as a pathognomonic symptom, would you say that changes in reality of the experiences but not of the concepts were more likely to occur in schizophrenia or less likely than in other conditions? In comparison with delirium or alcoholic hallucinosis or with organic dis-

eases, would the person with organic disease be
more likely than the schizophrenic to hear voices
but not believe they were real?

**Dr. Gottlieb:**  Yes.

**Dr. Malamud:**  So that really is not a pathognomonic
symptom of schizophrenia but it does occur. What
other special features here make us feel this is
schizophrenia?

**Dr. Gottlieb:**  The lack of interest in her ultimate outcome, the splitting of her emotional life, the splitting of her affect.

**Dr. Malamud:**  What are the most specific features of
schizophrenia? What are the primary symptoms?

**Dr. Gottlieb:**  The splitting of the affect or emotions
and withdrawal from the environment.

**Dr. Malamud:**  What do you notice about the associations here?

**Dr. Gottlieb:**  There is considerable difficulty in thought
at times. There were a few times when the associations seemed to be abnormal but usually her responses were fairly relevant to the questions. She did
seem to have some definite disturbance, as indicated
by her hesitancy, and at times her responses indicated that there was something disrupting her associations in schizophrenic fashion.

**Dr. Malamud:**  The most important feature is the fact
that the patient does not seem to be able to use language which actually expresses what she feels. That
was characteristic all through the interview here.
You can see that she actually wants to feel you, she
has no difficulty in finding words, but she cannot
find something which will adequately express what
she actually feels. "It's something different; I can't
explain." That is very typical of schizophrenia. One
of the most important underlying features is the as-
sociational disturbance. It is because of this disturbance that associations become short or
nonsensical. Apparently, there is an undercurrent
going on but at a level which does not lend itself to

logical expression in language. She also has hallucinations and paranoid ideas about being hypnotized,
what Bleuler calls accessory things. What do you
think about keeping her on, Dr. Weatherly?

**Dr. Weatherly:**    I do not know whether it would be worthwhile to attempt a discussion of these things further
or not. It seems to me that with this disturbance in
association, her own feeling of vagueness and the difficulty in attention which she has, continued work
with her would not greatly influence the course.

Her diagnosis was that of schizophrenia, hebephrenic type,
and she was transferred to the state hospital for further hospitalization. There was no psychiatric illness in the family.

In the short-term follow-up at the state hospital in March
1937, she was disturbed and had an exacerbation of her
hallucinations, and her behavior was characterized by silly
laughter and confusion. In April 1938, she was in the state
hospital on a semidisturbed ward. She was mute, her eyes
were closed, and she smiled when addressed. She was careless, postured, occasionally violent, and resistant to care.
Though she still wrote sensible letters, she was considered
to be mentally deteriorated.

# ▌ NNS

A 20-year-old, single woman was admitted August 9, 1940,
because of apathy and lack of spontaneous remarks. She
was irrelevant in her responses and unable to keep a job.
Her associations were considered loose and she was continually picking at her face.

She had always been a shy, retiring person, and these
traits had increased in the 2 years prior to admission. She
was attending college, and her academic work had become
poor by the fall of 1939. She developed a period of trem-
bling during which she was unable to talk, and she made
queer noises in her throat. When seen in the hospital, she
talked in a low voice, would only occasionally glance at the
examiner, and seemed dejected. She had definite ideas of

inferiority. On the ward she was quiet and withdrawn and did not talk spontaneously.

## Staff Meeting: August 20, 1940

Q:  Good morning, N.

A:  Good morning.

Q:  Take a seat.

A:  (Patient mumbled inaudibly without being questioned)

Q:  You have been talking out there and having a visit?

A:  Yes.

Q:  With whom?

A:  (Answer inaudible)

Q:  Did you have a nice visit with her?

A:  Yes.

Q:  Have you made friends with any of the girls on the ward?

A:  Not very much.

Q:  Don't you like them?

A:  Yes.

Q:  Are they nice to you?

A:  Yes.

Q:  What sort of things go on in the ward? Do people talk to you?

A:  Yes.

Q:  Do you get some work to do?

A:  Work on my crocheting and (inaudible) just whatever I can find to do.

Q:  And do you like it?

A:  Yes, I like it better.

Q:  When you first came here, didn't you like it?

A:  I didn't know at first.

Q:  Were you afraid?

A:  Sometimes I am.

Q:  What kind of things happen in the ward that make you afraid?

A:  Oh, afraid of not doing what I should—not doing it right.

**Q:** Do the nurses scold you?

**A:** No.

**Q:** Do they seem to be pleased with what you do?

**A:** Sometimes.

**Q:** What kind of mistakes do you make?

**A:** Oh, I don't try hard enough.

**Q:** Don't you want to do well?

**A:** I want to, but I don't always do it.

**Q:** You are bright and know what you ought to do.

**A:** I'm not smart enough.

**Q:** If you had something to do—like make a bed, you know how to do it?

**A:** Yes.

**Q:** And what keeps you from doing it well?

**A:** I can do that all right.

**Q:** In getting along with other people—do other people do things to your mind that make you think strange things?

**A:** No.

**Q:** Do things happen in your mind that make you afraid?

**A:** Yes, sometimes.

**Q:** Tell about that.

**A:** I think—

**Q:** What kinds of things happen in your mind?

**A:** When I think I should do something and don't know what to do. I'm not doing something that I should— I'm not trying hard.

**Q:** Do people make your mind think things?

**A:** Oh, sometimes.

**Q:** Do you have strange thoughts sometimes that trouble you?

**A:** I always go around in circles.

**Q:** And when you go in circles, what sort of thoughts come?

**A:** Things I have already done.

**Q:** Do you hear people talking to you sometimes when they are not there?

**A:** No.

Q: At night when you are alone in bed, can you tell what people are thinking about you?

A: (Inaudible)—standing close.

Q: You felt as if somebody were standing close?

A: Yes.

Q: Were they people that you knew?

A: (Answer inaudible)

Q: Did they seem to be friendly people?

A: (Inaudible)—suspicious.

Q: You were or they were?

A: (Answer inaudible)

Q: Do you think they meant to do something harmful to you?

A: I don't know.

Q: Why is it you are here in the hospital?

A: To get better.

Q: To get better of what?

A: It is to straighten things out.

Q: To straighten what, you?

A: Oh, work—(inaudible)

Q: Yes, all right—that will be enough this morning. You may go back, N., to the ward.

## Staff Meeting: October 15, 1940

Q: Come in N.

A: Good morning.

Q: Tell us what you are thinking about.

A: I was waiting for you to ask me questions.

Q: Are you thinking about something interesting? What do you like to think about?

A: I like to think about how I can get along.

Q: Are you happy?

A: No.

Q: You would like to succeed in the world wouldn't you?

A: Yes.

Q: Is there any reason why you shouldn't?

A: No, I don't think so.

Q: You think there is no reason.

**A:** No.

**Q:** You have gone to school and college and know a good many things.

**A:** No . . . no.

**Q:** Have you forgotten much?

**A:** Don't use—I mean studies. Don't use studies very much. I don't know much. I don't use it much.

**Q:** When you try to remember things that you have studied or read, do you find some difficulty?

**A:** Sometimes, I don't always. I didn't always study so good. When I did study good, I wouldn't remember some.

**Q:** Is it good English grammar to say "I study good"? What ought you say?

**A:** Study well.

**Q:** And history—do you remember anything about Grover Cleveland?

**A:** He was a President, that is all.

**Q:** And what sort of an impression do you have about him? Was he successful or unsuccessful?

**A:** I don't know. I never thought about it.

**Q:** Do you remember anything about Abraham Lincoln's boyhood?

**A:** I do a little.

**Q:** Tell me what you remember.

**A:** He studied a lot, lived with his parents in a log cabin, and he used to sleep upstairs, no he used to sleep— he used to think over things the people talked about; he used to ponder over them.

**Q:** What do you admire him most for? I mean, what qualities to you admire most in him?

**A:** I never thought about it before. I suppose—he was democratic (inaudible)—Oh—(inaudible)—Oh (inaudible)—and straight forward.

**Q:** What kind of people do you admire most now?

**A:** I don't know.[5]

**Q:** What qualities do you admire most in people?

---

[5] *Note.*    Inaudible, but, I believe, "mind their own business."

A: (Inaudible)—Oh—(inaudible)—Oh (inaudible)—and thoughtful.

Q: If you could add some qualities to yourself, what would you wish most for?

A: I don't know.

Q: Your parents?

A: Well (inaudible)—some obedience to (inaudible)

Q: To be successful in the world, what would you like most to add to your qualities to help you succeed?

A: Get along—oh, fit myself to do outside work well—I don't know. (Inaudible)

Q: Mix with people did you say?

A: Yes. (inaudible)—still.

Q: Do you feel that people like you as much as you want them to?

A: I never thought of that.

Q: You never thought about that? Most people do, don't they?

A: Yes.

Q: Are you feeling well? Are you worrying over anything?

A: No.

Q: Do you notice that you keep your eyes partly shut?

A: Yes.

Q: Why is that?

A: I don't know.

Q: Do you feel embarrassed at being before us here? Don't you enjoy being here?

A: I don't know.

Q: Isn't it nice to be before a lot of people, to have them look at you and pay attention to you?

A: (Inaudible)

Q: All right—that will be enough this morning.

## Staff Discussion Following the Interview

**Dr. Emmons:**   I feel that the diagnosis "schizophrenia" should be continued. I am not entirely sure of the sub-group. The previous diagnosis was "schizophrenia, unclassified."

**Dr. Woods:**   Does anyone feel much doubt as to what this is as to subclass?

**Dr. Miller:**   It is probably hebephrenia, with all this grimacing and smiling. Is that acceptable to any others? (Majority agree.) We will put it down then as "schizophrenia, hebephrenia."

**Dr. Emmons:**   The home situation is not too satisfactory. Yet, I hesitate to suggest state hospitalization because I think that the patient can get along on the outside so long as she is somewhat protected. The family of course are willing to have her at home, and I think she can get by there even though it is not too satisfactory.

**Dr. Woods:**   From what we know of the home, Dr. Ruilmann, what would you advise?

**Dr. Ruilmann:**   I'm afraid I don't know much about the home.

**Dr. Woods:**   The father is a drunkard and the family is in low economic circumstances. The mother is a neurotic. Does she interfere with the patient?

**Dr. Emmons:**   She is somewhat solicitous about her and has a tendency to worry.

**Dr. Woods:**   The question would be between state hospitalization, which would possibly be better for the patient, or living at home to avoid the unhappy thought of having her at the hospital. Being in a state hospital wouldn't bother her very much. It is just a question of which type of protection would bring her out more.

**Dr. Emmons:**   She has written several letters even recently that she would be sorry to leave here, her room and the friends that she has made here. So as you say, I don't think state hospitalization would trouble her.

**Dr. Gottlieb:**   I think for this patient, state hospitalization would be best in view of the poor family situation.

**Dr. Miller:**   I am wondering whether it wouldn't be better for the patient to be in a state hospital, even if

the family were a good one. I know of three girls
with schizophrenia who have done extremely well at
Mt. Pleasant with this level of intelligence. They do
put patients like this on the parole board, and they
get into hospital occupation.

**Dr. Woods:**    I think it would be better for her to go to a
state hospital. At home, there would be a great deal
of competition, or being compared with others, and
they are bound to say, "Why don't you do so and so?"
Let us recommend state hospitalization, and if they
greatly desire her at home, we are willing to let
them try it, but let us advise hospitalization, and
send her there if they wish us to do so. The patient's
diagnosis was schizophrenia, hebephrenic type, and
the recommendation was for state hospitalization.

She was given a course of insulin coma treatment with little
improvement. It was advised that she be sent to a state hospital but was discharged on October 21, 1940, to her father.

The family history was positive for mental disease. A sister was a psychiatric patient in both the Iowa Psychiatric
Hospital and the state hospital for a total of 1 year. The
father was alcoholic and had a nervous breakdown at age
18.

Although the father did not want her at a state hospital,
by October 1940 (a few days after discharge) she was sent
to a state hospital. In March 1941, they said that she was
mute, had to be tube fed, and had been restrained. She
spent her entire day in idleness. By April 1942, a report
from the state hospital stated that she gazed into the distance, was depressed, was difficult to draw into conversation, but oriented. Her course had been unfavorable, and
for the first year she was violent, combative, untidy, and had
to be tube fed. She refused to talk. She was disinterested,
catatonic, and spent her time in idleness. That was the last
report in the short-term follow-up.

The previous interviews are from representative patients
of the Iowa 500. Their histories, interviews, and short-term
follow-up are typical of the patients with schizophrenia,

bipolar disorder, and unipolar disorder that were admitted to a psychiatric hospital before the advent of effective treatment. Because of the active therapies that are now available, it is difficult to assess the natural histories of these disorders in modern patients. Today, however, though the symptoms and course have been altered, many aspects of the clinical picture described in the case studies and interviews still remain.

# Chapter 7

## Follow-Up of Untreated Patients

*Course of the Illness Unaffected by Effective Therapy*

"Five years have past, five summers"

—William Wordsworth,
"Lines, Composed a Few
Miles Above Tintern Abbey"

The short-term chart follow-up of the Iowa 500 is particularly important in that it covers a period when no treatment was available. There was no electroconvulsive therapy (ECT), no antidepressant drug therapy, no lithium, no neuroleptic treatment, and, at that time, lobotomies were not being performed. Thus, the first follow-up is pristine in terms of having no contamination from treatment. As noted previously, 315 patients given a clinical diagnosis of schizophrenia were excluded from the study. However, these patients had the same kind of detailed follow-up data in their charts, and, in evaluating the unipolar depressive, bipolar, and schizophrenic patients, we also made a comparison with this group, which we termed the "schizophreniform

131

group." This group appeared to be schizophrenic but did not specifically meet the criteria and, consequently, was separated from the schizophrenic patients who were diagnosed according to rigorous standards. Certainly, it was conceivable that a large number of these patients were schizophrenic, but, as they did not meet the research criteria, we thought they might have a somewhat different kind of outcome than those schizophrenic patients who did meet the criteria.

It was the style and tradition of the Iowa State Psychopathic Hospital to obtain follow-up information on each discharged patient. The social service department sent out questionnaires at 6-month and 1-year intervals to parents or other family members, and telephone follow-ups were often made as well. Physicians in the community as well as physicians at other psychiatric institutions were contacted for their input. Often, discharged patients came back to see their physician at the Psychopathic Hospital where additional information could be obtained from personal interviews.

As the follow-up information was reported on a totally separate section of the chart, it was possible to evaluate the subsequent course of a patient's illness without knowledge of the specific intake information. However, it was usually evident whether the patient's diagnosis had been that of affective disorder or schizophrenia. On the other hand, the follow-up evaluations of the 515 charts that carried a clinical diagnosis of schizophrenia were blind because the reviewers did not know who met the strict diagnostic criteria.

The sources of follow-up information in percentages for bipolar illness, unipolar depression, schizophrenia, and schizophreniform psychosis were as follows: No follow-up information was available on 7%, 5%, 4%, and 6%, respectively. An interview with the patient was available on 17%, 16%, 17%, and 20%, respectively. Information was gleaned from a friend or relative in 29%, 33%, 25%, and 26%, and a letter from a subsequent hospital or physician was available in 44%, 45%, 53%, and 47%. Other sources of follow-up information only accounted for 1%–3% (Morrison et al. 1972).

The following categories of recovery were used:

1. **Well.**   These patients were asymptomatic and back to their usual occupation. The rating was dependent on a relative, friend, or physician who knew the individual patient well enough to assess him or her and state that he or she appeared completely normal and was back to his or her usual self, functioning in an ordinary and usual capacity. The patients may have had subsequent episodes of illness, but they were known to have become completely recovered.
2. **Social recovery.**   Although these patients had returned to their usual occupation and were not hospitalized, they had residual symptoms.
3. **Ill without recovery.**   These patients were continuously symptomatic and functioned poorly regardless of whether they were in or out of a mental institution.
4. **Never recovered and deteriorated.**   These patients had difficulty communicating and showed inability to care for themselves and inability to work; they were incapacitated.

Some patients were known to be socially recovered, functioning outside of the hospital, although their current mental status was unknown; other patients were known to be outside of the hospital, although it was not known whether they were medically or socially recovered.

The mean follow-up for the unipolar depressive patients was 4.3 years; for patients with bipolar disorder, 2.2 years; for schizophrenic patents, 2.6 years; and for the patients with schizophreniform psychosis, 3.2 years. Table 7–1 presents the percentage of each outcome category after the short-term follow-up. The numbers are smaller than the original sample size because follow-up information was not available on all subjects. Some percentage totals are greater than 100 because patients could be classified in two categories. Thus, a patient who was deteriorated was generally rated as ill without remission. The findings are notable because over half of the patients with affective disorder showed total recovery at some point in the short term follow-up, although about 20% continued to be ill without remission. On the other hand, only 8% of the schizophrenic patients were likely to recover—about one-third as many as those patients with schizophreniform psychosis ($P = .001$). At short-term follow-up, three-quarters of the schizophrenic patients, but only one-half of the schizophreniform patients ($P = .01$), were ill.

Table 7–2 presents the recovery according to the length of follow-up. This is the proportion of patients who had been totally recovered at a specific point in time, whether or not they were ill at last follow-up. In addition, Figure 7–1 presents these recovery data graphically. There are no significant differences between the bipolar and the unipolar groups at any point in time. Within 10–20 years, almost all patients that had affective disorders had shown a complete recovery. In the case of the schizophrenic and the schizophreniform patients, the picture is different. None of the schizophrenic patients were recovered by 6 months as compared with the affective disorder patients of whom about one-quarter were well at some point. By 2–3 years, however, 12% of the schizophrenic patients were considered

**Table 7–1.**    Outcome at short-term follow-up from medical records

| Diagnostic group | Recovered ever (%) | Social recovery (%) | Ill without remission (%) | Deteriorated (%) |
|---|---|---|---|---|
| Bipolar affective disorder ($n = 87$) | 54 | 51 | 21 | 0 |
| Unipolar affective disorder ($n = 202$) | 59 | 61 | 20 | 2 |
| Schizophrenia ($n = 183$) | 8 | 19 | 78 | 13 |
| Schizophreniform psychosis ($n = 284$) | 22 | 40 | 51 | 12 |

*Source.*    Adapted from Morrison et al. 1972.

**Table 7–2** Proportion of patients recovered according to number followed for a specific length of time

| | Length of follow-up | | | | | | | | |
|---|---|---|---|---|---|---|---|---|---|
| | 1–6 months | | 1 year | | 2–3 years | | 5 years | | 10–20 years | |
| Diagnostic group | n | recovered (%) | n | recovered (%) | n | recovered (%) | n | recovered (%) | n | recovered (%) |
| Bipolar | 22 | (27) | 36 | (47) | 13 | (69) | 10 | (90) | 6 | (100) |
| Unipolar | 38 | (29) | 58 | (43) | 23 | (57) | 42 | (76) | 41 | (95) |
| Schizophrenia | 34 | (0) | 61 | (3) | 58 | (12) | 14 | (14) | 16 | (19) |
| Schizophreniform | 42 | (2) | 76 | (13) | 96 | (30) | 47 | (32) | 23 | (35) |

Source. Adapted from Morrison et al. 1972.

recovered. This then stabilized; in the 10- to 20-year period, about 19% were considered to have recovered.

The slope with the recovery curve for the schizophreniform patients is similar to that for the affective disorders during the first 2 years of follow-up (Figure 7–1). Subsequently, few patients recover, and the curve is identical in slope with that of the schizophrenic patients. This suggests that some of the schizophreniform patients bore a considerable relationship to the affective disorder patients but that the majority were schizophrenic in nature.

Each patient known to be continuously hospitalized at a given time interval is also scored positively at all earlier follow-up periods in Table 7–3. None of the patients were continuously hospitalized at the Iowa Psychopathic Hospital. They had been transferred to other institutions and were counted as continuously hospitalized for the remainder of their confinement. Data are presented in Figure 7–2 in a more dramatic fashion showing that by the second year of follow-up fewer than 5% of the affective disorder patients remained continuously hospitalized, but

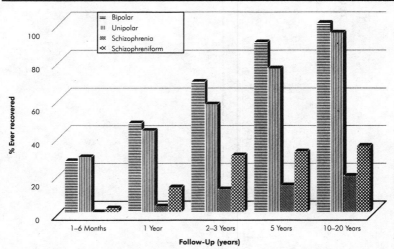

**Figure 7–1.** Patient recovery according to length of follow-up. *Source.* Adapted from Morrison et al. 1972.

one-fifth of the schizophrenic patients remained continuously hospitalized after 5 years. Though the data are few at 10 years, the continuous hospitalization rate seems to have stabilized for the schizophrenic patients. Patients with schizophreniform psychosis are separate from both the affective disorder and the schizophrenic patients. Chronic hospitalization was not seen in any more than one-quarter of the schizophreniform patients, and, by 5 or 10 years, only 5% have remained chronically hospitalized. The differences between these groups are all significant.

Again, it should be noted that evaluation of follow-up in the schizophrenic versus the schizophreniform patients was blind, as there was no way to know which of these patients, all of whom received a hospital diagnosis of schizophrenia, did or did not fill the research criteria. Likewise, it was not known by the raters into which original category the patient had been placed at follow-up, meaning, for instance, that an individual rating at 10 years was blind to the rating at 6 months or 1 year. In a sense, this blindness is a testimony to the validity of the selection criteria. The data show minor differences in outcome between the types of affective disorders but none reach significance.

Table 7–4 presents course differences between bipolar and unipolar patients. It is important to note that the polarity is

**Table 7–3.** Patients continuously hospitalized since index admission according to length of follow-up

| Length of follow-up | Bipolar n Hosp (%) | Unipolar n Hosp (%) | Schizo- phrenic n Hosp (%) | Schizophreni- form n Hosp (%) |
|---|---|---|---|---|
| 1–6 months | 92 (12) | 210 (14) | 190 (40) | 293 (22) |
| 1 year | 66 (9) | 170 (11) | 150 (39) | 248 (21) |
| 2 years | 30 (3) | 107 (2) | 88 (28) | 168 (12) |
| 3 years | 20 (0) | 97 (2) | 61 (25) | 137 (12) |
| 5 years | 16 (0) | 83 (1) | 30 (20) | 70 (6) |
| 10 years | 6 (0) | 41 (0) | 16 (19) | 22 (5) |

*Source.* Adapted from Morrison et al. 1972.

based on final diagnostic assessment after long-term follow-up, which resulted in 22 of the 225 depressive patients becoming bipolar. One other aspect of the course has to do with the pre-index and discharge variables, such as bipolar patients being considerably younger at index than the unipolar patients, and their median age at onset also being different. From onset to index, the bipolar patients have been ill a shorter period of time, but they have more episodes prior to admission. Thus, 52% of the bipolar patients had one or more episodes prior to admission, whereas 37% of the unipolar patients experienced a similar background. At discharge, both are equally likely to be markedly improved or well, and it should be noted that this level of improvement at time of hospitalization discharge may not be relevant to having an increased number of episodes in the bipolar group during the follow-up. Notably, in bipolar patients, those patients who manifested psychotic symptoms (delusions and hallucinations) had a later age at onset.

Other points are important in the early evaluation of follow-up material. The original 225 unipolar depressive patients were

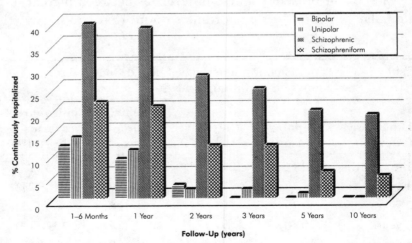

**Figure 7–2.**    Patient follow-up of those who were continuously hospitalized.
*Source.*    Adapted from Morrison et al. 1973.

evaluated specifically in regard to the chart follow-up (Winokur and Morrison 1973). Of the original 225 depressive patients, 9 became bipolar in the course of the chart follow-up; 8 were male, and 1 was female. This preponderance of males ($P$ = .025) occurred despite the fact that, of the original 225, females outnumbered males 124 to 101. In the chart follow-up of 1 month to 20 years, 4.2% had changed from unipolar to bipolar. Of the nine who became manic, eight became manic within 3 years of index admission. Of the 35 patients followed-up in the chart for 10–20 years, only 1 (2.8%) became manic. Thus, in order to study a group of depressive patients, one must recognize that some proportion will, at some point, change from unipolar to bipolar. Within the first 3 years of the study, however, this percentage is small. Nevertheless, as time passes, other unipolar depressive patients do convert to bipolarity, which can introduce a substantial error in diagnosis. Stability of diagnosis, therefore, was a very important factor to consider in this study.

**Table 7–4.**   Course differences in bipolar versus unipolar depressive patients

|  | Bipolar[a] (n = 122) | Unipolar[a] (n = 203) |
|---|---|---|
| Median age at index[b] | 30–33 | 46–45 |
| Median age at onset[b] | 24–29 | 37 |
| One or more episodes prior to admission, n (%) | 63 (52) | 89 (37) |
| Marked improvement or well at discharge, n (%) | 37 (30) | 74 (36) |
| Complete recovery during follow-up, n (%) | 59 (48) | 108 (53) |

[a]Based on long-term follow-up assessments, 22 of the original 225 depressive patients (unipolar) became bipolar.
[b]First age is for nonpsychotic patients; second age is for patients with psychoses.

As we assessed the follow-up in the unipolar depressed patients, we were particularly interested in the relationship of three variables to follow-up: age at onset, age at index, and gender. To accomplish this, it was necessary to divide the unipolar patients into six groups (Winokur 1973b, Winokur 1974b). These groups included males and females divided into those that were young (younger than 40) with an early onset (younger than 40), those who had an early onset but were older than 40 at time of index admission, and those who were older than 40 for both onset and index admission. The patients who were evaluated were the 216 unipolar patients that remained after 9 patients had become bipolar in the follow-up.

For the total follow-up time (6 months to 20 years), we evaluated the number of episodes and also the question of chronicity, which was defined as being ill from time of index admission to time of last follow-up. Chronicity included patients who made a social recovery but who continued to have subsequent symptoms, as well as those who were both socially and symptomatically unrecovered. It was clear that males had more episodes per year at follow-up than did females. Also, males were more likely to have one or more subsequent episodes than females. Neither age at onset nor age at index admission was related to the number of episodes in follow-up. There was no significant difference between males and females regarding chronicity at the time of follow-up. Age at index admission indicated that older patients were more likely to be chronic at the time of follow-up than younger patients, although age at onset was not related to chronicity. If one evaluates a more substantial follow-up (2–20 years), it becomes quite apparent that females are more likely to be chronic than males. For women, age at onset is not related to the development of chronicity over this longer period of time; however, age itself is related to chronicity, with older women showing more chronicity. Some data suggested that, as the males became older, they had more episodes per year at follow-up time. Likewise, if one looked at the substantial follow-up of 2–20 years, it was clear that the group that was most likely to be chronic were females who were older than

40 at index admission; however, age at onset did not predict chronicity in these female depressive patients. It was also noteworthy that, in patients who were followed for 1 year or more, 44 were chronic at the end of the follow-up period and 102 were not chronic. Only 2% of the chronic patients had an alcoholic father whereas 15% of the remitted patients had alcoholic fathers, indicating that family history predicted chronicity. In other words, the presence of alcoholism in a father predicted an illness that remitted in 13 months or less.

Such findings as these are important for two reasons. If chronicity is more frequent in females than in males, a natural history aspect of the course must be considered in studies of treatment efficacy. Because of the increased risk for chronicity in females, one might ask whether some antidepressant regimens are better than others. A study of antidepressants performed by the British Medical Research Council offered evidence that males responded better than females to tricyclic medication (Medical Research Council 1969). Furthermore, increased remission rate in males may be, to some extent, due to the fact that they are more likely to have subsequent episodes than females and are also more likely to have spontaneous recoveries.

A second area of usefulness for course data is in the separation of homogeneous or autonomous disease groups. Using specific criteria for depression, and, in the absence of a manic episode, one can be reasonably certain to have a 90%–95% yield of unipolar depressive patients for follow-up. It is entirely possible that differences in course are relevant to differences in diagnosis and that some patients with very specific subtype diagnoses in affective disorder have very specific courses. This is still a matter of considerable importance in clinical studies of depression at present.

The natural history of the untreated psychiatric patient is a matter of great significance to the clinician. It provides a benchmark against which all treatment efforts must be measured. The salient features of the short-term follow-up of these untreated patients are essentially as follows: Both bipolar and unipolar affective disorder patients recover over time in the majority of cases. This recovery is reflected by both the absence of clinical symptomatology and the recovery of social productivity. This is different in patients with clearly diagnosed schizophrenia where a small minority ever achieve either social recovery or recovery from the symptoms. Clear chronicity is far more frequent in the schizophrenic patients, and deterioration is mainly seen in these patients. Patients who have schizophreniform psychosis show symptoms that are similar to those of schizophrenic patients but have a relatively acute onset. This probably reflects a mixture of schizophrenic and affective disorder patients. The majority of untreated bipolar and unipolar patients take between 2 to 3 years for recovery. By a 10- to 25-year follow-up, almost all have at least had some period of recovery. Chronic hospitalization reflects recovery. Schizophrenic patients are far more likely to be chronically hospitalized than are the affective disorder patients. In a short period of time, approximately 5% of unipolar patients go on to bipolarity. Bipolar patients are more likely younger at index admission and younger at onset of their illness than unipolar patients, and they are more likely to have multiple episodes prior to admission. Complete recovery occurs at some time equally in bipolar and unipolar patients. Such clear-cut differences as are presented in this chapter support the fact that bipolar affective disorder, unipolar depression, and schizophrenia are autonomous illnesses.

# Chapter 8

# Families

*Familial Psychiatric Illnesses Obtained by*
*Systematically Obtained Family Histories*

"... each unhappy family is unhappy in
its own way."

—Leo Tolstoy, *Anna Karenina*

Like the previous chapter, the data presented here reflect a systematic evalu-
ation of the medical records. The family histories of the manic,
depressive, and schizophrenic patients had been obtained in an
organized fashion and had been recorded in the early 1930s
and 1940s by social workers and psychiatrists working in the
hospital. A family history is to be differentiated from a family
study, the latter being personal examination of relatives at risk.
In the case of the family history, the patient and perhaps
another relative or friend is questioned about the presence of
psychiatric illness in the family. Some cases are certainly lost
by the family history method. Winokur and colleagues (1969)
showed that there were a substantial number of patients who
were positive by interview but negative by family history. These
would then be false negatives. Certainly, the personal examination should be considered the gold standard for diagnosis.

There were virtually no people who were positive by family history and negative by personal examination so that there were almost no false positives. Although some cases are lost by the family history method, Thompson and co-workers (1982) have shown that the specificity of diagnoses is acceptable. What one does lose is a certain amount of sensitivity since not as many cases of ill family members are picked up as might be ascertained by using material from all sources (i.e., personal interviews, family history, and record perusal).

The family histories of the patients in the Iowa 500 included lengthy descriptions of the personalities and mental illnesses of parents, siblings, and children, and they frequently contained similar material about both sets of grandparents, maternal and paternal aunts and uncles, and even more remote relatives. Some of the probands had relatives who had been admitted to the Iowa Psychopathic Hospital, and these records were examined. It was the practice between 1934 and 1944 to obtain records on relatives who had psychiatric admissions at other hospitals. All of the family history data were duplicated, omitting any reference to the patient's sex, diagnosis, symptoms, year of admission, or outcome of illness and were evaluated blindly by one of the people involved in the research (Winokur et al. 1972).

The blindness in making the diagnoses was quite effective, although in a few cases (probably less than 10), it was possible to read the family history material and determine the diagnosis of the proband. The major diagnoses that were made were those of schizophrenia, affective disorder, and alcoholism. Schizophrenia was diagnosed in a relative if the illness began before age 40 and went on to either chronic hospitalization or chronic social incapacity. Evidence of marked affective symptoms placed the relative into the category of an undiagnosed psychosis. In order for schizophrenia to be diagnosed in a family member, there had to be some evidence of bizarre behavior, delusional thinking, or seclusiveness over a long period of time. If a relative suffered from an illness with common affective symptoms from which he or she recovered without significant personality defect, he or she was considered to have an affective disorder. This diagnosis was made regardless of whether hospitalization for his or her illness was involved or not. In a sense then, the differentiation between schizophrenia and affective disorder was based essentially on the presence or absence of a remitting illness.

Sometimes the family histories included diagnoses made by hospitals or physicians, which were usually accepted unless there was some reason to believe that the diagnoses did not fit the criteria given above. When criteria were equivocal, the diagnosis of undiagnosed psychosis or undiagnosed minor psychiatric illness was made.

Alcoholism was diagnosed if the family history noted that a relative had problems because of excessive alcohol intake or if it was noted that the relative was considered a pathological drinker.

The family history data are those concerned with the original selection of probands (i.e., 200 schizophrenic, 100 bipolar, 225 unipolar depressive patients). Morbid risks were calculated for depression and schizophrenia for parents and siblings of the three groups of index cases. Morbid risks (or disease expectancy) is the probability that a relative will show the disease in question at some time during his or her life if he or she survives the risk period (manifestation period) for the disease. The Weinberg Short method for correcting for age distribution was used. This method approximates the more sophisticated methodology used today for estimating morbidity risks. In this method, the number of relatives who have not yet entered the age of risk and half the number of those who are between the upper and lower limits of the age of risk are deducted from the total number of the class of relatives. For depression, these limits were taken as between 15 and 60 years of age, corresponding to the ages at onset of the probands of the study that had affective illnesses. For schizophrenia, limits were between 15 and 40 years of age. Anybody older than those ages was counted in full, whereas anybody within those ages was counted as one-half. If the relatives were younger than age 15, they were not counted at all. The number at risk for suicide was considered the same as the number at risk for affective disorder. Comparisons of groups were made using chi-square method with Yates correction for small numbers.

At the time of entry into the study, schizophrenic, manic, and depressive patients had median ages of 27, 30, and 45 years, respectively. The schizophrenic patients had 3.1 siblings per proband, manic patients had 3.6, and the depressive patients had 4.3. Schizophrenic patients, being younger, had more siblings younger than age 15, and we did not report siblings younger than age 15.

In the familial illness estimation, few parents in any of the three groups were unknown: none in schizophrenia, two in the manic group, and three in the depressed group. Undiagnosed psychoses were seen in seven parents in each group.

Table 8–1 presents the risks for schizophrenia in the relatives of the proband groups. The risk for schizophrenia in the relatives of schizophrenic patients was significantly higher ($P$ = .005) than the risks in the combined group of affective disorder probands. Risks for affective disorder are shown in Table 8–2. No attempt was made to separate family members with bipolar disorder from those with unipolar disorder in this section of the family history comparisons. A perusal of Table 8–2 shows a clear increase in morbid risks for affective disorder in the family members of both the manic and depressive probands. What is particularly interesting is that the morbid risks for affective disorder in the parents and siblings of schizophrenic patients is actually higher than the morbid risks for schizophrenia in these family members. This is consistent with the findings of psychiatric disorders among relatives of surgical control subjects (Tsuang et al. 1984). The morbid risks for mania and depression in the relatives of control subjects was 7.6% as compared with the morbid risk of schizophrenia of .6%. It is probable that though the morbid risks for affective disorder are higher in the relatives of schizophrenic probands than are the morbid risks for schizophrenia, this high risk for affective disorder is simply a reflection of the normal population frequency.

**Table 8–1.** Morbid risks for schizophrenia in parents and siblings of manic, depressive, and schizophrenic probands: blind family history comparison

|  | Schizophrenic | At risk | Morbid risk (%) |
|---|---|---|---|
| Schizophrenic probands |  |  |  |
| Parents | 7 | 384 | 1.82 |
| Siblings | 6 | 233 | 2.58 |
| Parents/siblings | 13 | 617 | 2.11 |
| Manic probands |  |  |  |
| Parents | 1 | 193 | .52 |
| Siblings | 4 | 241 | 1.66 |
| Depressive probands |  |  |  |
| Parents | 1 | 426 | .23 |
| Siblings | 4 | 802 | .49 |
| All affective disorder probands |  |  |  |
| Parents | 2 | 619 | .32 |
| Siblings | 8 | 1,043 | .77 |
| Parents/siblings | 10 | 1,662 | .62 |

*Note.* Differences: parents and siblings of patients who were manic and depressives versus parents and siblings of schizophrenic patients, $P < .005$.
*Source.* Adapted from Winokur et al. 1972

Suicide in parents and siblings of schizophrenic and affective disorder probands was significantly different ($P= .025$). As opposed to 3% of the relatives of affective disorder probands, 1.1% of the relatives of schizophrenic probands committed suicide.

In a blind assessment of "minor illnesses," some effort was made to record neuroses, personality disorders, and significant nervousness in the parents of the three groups probands. Of 400 parents of schizophrenic probands, 79 (20%) were considered to have some evidence of a "minor" psychiatric illness. Of the 650 parents of the affective disorder probands (mania, bipolar, and unipolar patients), 71 (11%) had evidence of these kinds of problems. The difference is highly significant. This suggests the possibility that schizophrenia manifests itself in incomplete forms of psychopathology that do not meet criteria for schizo-phrenia. These "minor illnesses" are hard to define in a family history study.

The family history analyses separate schizophrenia from the affective disorders well. There are, however, a series of other findings that are also relevant to the family history. In Tables 8–1 and 8–2, it was clear that affective disorder was more likely found in families of affective disorder patients, and schizophrenia was more likely found in the families of schizophrenic patients. We evaluated this in extended families as well as first-degree relatives. A family history of affective disorder, schizophrenia, and alcoholism was seen respectively in 17.5%, 6.5%, and 15% of the families of 200 schizophrenic patients and 18.4%, 3.1%, and 5.9% in the families of the 325 affective disor-

**Table 8–2.**  Morbid risks for affective disorder in parents and siblings of manic, depressive, and schizophrenic probands: blind family history comparison

|  | Affective disorder | At risk | Morbid risk (%) |
|---|---|---|---|
| Schizophrenic probands | | | |
| Parents | 20 | 274 | 7.30 |
| Siblings | 12 | 310 | 3.88 |
| Parents/siblings | 32 | 584 | 5.50 |
| Manic probands | | | |
| Parents | 15 | 145 | 10.30 |
| Siblings | 22 | 183 | 12.00 |
| Depressive probands | | | |
| Parents | 45 | 350 | 12.80 |
| Siblings | 78 | 509 | 15.30 |
| All affective disorder probands | | | |
| Parents | 60 | 495 | 12.10 |
| Siblings | 100 | 692 | 14.50 |
| Parents/siblings | 160 | 1,187 | 13.50 |

*Note.*  Differences: parents of manic and depressive patients versus parents of schizophrenic patients, $P < .05$; siblings of manic and depressive patients versus siblings of schizophrenic patients, $P < .0005$.
*Source.*  Adapted from Winokur et al. 1972.

der patients (Winokur 1975a). The extended families of the schizophrenic patients were more than twice as likely to show schizophrenia than the extended families of the affective disorder patients. The difference between the extended families on the variable of alcoholism was also highly significant ($P = .0005$). Thus, the same findings that one gets from the family history of primary relatives are found when one evaluates the extended family. In this case, any single family could be counted only once even if it had many members with affective disorder in it, and, consequently, the methodology does not lend itself to a particularly good separation of diagnoses on the basis of a family history of depression (Winokur 1975a).

## Relationship of Clinical Factors With Familial Subtypes of Depression

One possibility of solving the problem of heterogeneity within the affective disorders is to classify according to a specific family history. As an example, this is possible between bipolar and unipolar illness. Bipolar patients are more likely to have a positive family history of mania as well as a larger family history of affective disorder in general than are unipolar depressive patients. The family history, therefore, is related to a particular kind of clinical picture, namely the presence of manic excitement in the proband (Angst and Perris 1968; Winokur and Clayton 1967). In an effort to separate familial subtypes of unipolar depression, certain types of family history may be relevant. Winokur and associates (1971) suggested that one type of depression was associated with a family history of alcoholism. This type of depression is called depression spectrum disease. It is defined by the presence of alcoholism in a first-degree family member, usually a male. Depression spectrum disease probands may have depression in the family but no mania. Depression spectrum patients are separated from other types of depressive patients who may also be subdivided by family history. Familial pure depressive disease is a depression in an individual who has a family history of depression, no mania, and no alcoholism. Sporadic depressive disease is an illness where family history of the depressive proband shows no evidence of depression, alcoholism, or mania. The data from the Iowa 500 have been useful in evaluating this kind of familial subtyping. Winokur and colleagues (1973) evaluated the 225 original unipolar depressive patients in the Iowa 500. Early onset patients were more likely to have a family history of affective disorder, and early onset females in particular were more likely to have a family history of alcoholism in a male parent. In that evaluation, suicides were more frequently seen in parents of early onset patients, and early onset depressive illness was associated with more frequent episodes of illness prior to the index admission. Thus, there is an association between an early onset of illness, being female, and having a different kind of a course. Such data back up the concept of at least two types of depressive illness: one is that of depression spectrum disease and the other of pure depressive disease. The latter group may be divided into pure (familial) or sporadic depressive disease. Note that the names of the familial diseases are relevant to a specific kind of family background, mainly associated with the presence or absence of alcoholism or affective disorder (Winokur et al. 1973).

Also relevant to a familial separation of diseases was another finding. Chronic depression in the female is associated with a specific family history. The validity in a familial subtyping of depression is supported by the finding that the presence of an alcoholic father in the family reliably predicted against chronic depression. Chronicity was defined as continuous illness for 1 or more years after index admission and an individual was considered chronic if he or she did not recover from the symptoms even if a social recovery occurred. Of course, if the patient were both symptomatically and socially unrecovered, he or she was also considered chronic. Of 44 chronic patients in the Iowa 500, in the short-term follow-up, only 1%–2% had an alcoholic father, but, in those patients who were not chronic (i.e., had remitted prior to a year after index admission), 15% had alcoholic fathers

(Winokur 1974b). This suggests some validity in a familial subtyping of depression.

Another finding that supports the validity of a familial subtyping had to do with the duration of illness prior to hospitalization in depressive patients. Onset was defined as duration of illness prior to index admission. Manic patients were far more likely to have an acute onset when defined this way (Winokur 1976). Of equal importance was the fact that patients with a family history of alcoholism in a first-degree relative were much less likely than other depressive patients to have an acute onset of their illness. When unipolar depressive patients were separated into those who had a family history of alcoholism and those who had no family history of alcoholism (matched for sex and age at index admission), the depression spectrum group was much less likely to have an acute onset than the matched group. Thus, only 3% of the depression spectrum group had an onset within a month of illness, but 12% of the matched group (no family history of alcoholism) had an onset within a month. Twice as many of the matched group—37%—had an onset within 1–3 months when compared with the depression spectrum group—19%. Thus, the lack of an acute onset and a family history of alcoholism appear to coexist together.

## Psychotic Symptomatology in Bipolar and Unipolar Affective Illness

Bipolar and unipolar patients, respectively, were separated into psychotic and nonpsychotic subtypes (Winokur 1984). The bipolar patients numbered 122 and, thus, encompassed those who changed from unipolarity to bipolarity over the long follow-up; the unipolar patients numbered 203. Hallucinations and motor symptoms were more common in the bipolar patients. Ten percent of the 122 bipolar patients had motor symptoms such as tics and grimaces, but only 2% of the unipolar patients had these symptoms. Auditory hallucinations were more com-

mon in the bipolar patients (14% versus 6%) as were visual hallucinations (9% versus 1%). The bipolar patients were separated
into those who had psychotic symptoms and those who did not.
This was also done for the unipolar patients. Seventy-eight
(64%) of the bipolar and 113 (57%) of the 203 unipolar patients had psychotic symptoms. These psychotic symptoms
were both mood congruent and mood incongruent symptoms
such as passivity, symbolism, persecutory delusions, and
thought broadcasting. Fifty-one percent of the bipolar and 46%
of the unipolar patients had persecutory delusions. Primary delusions or symbolism was seen in 5% and 7% of bipolar and
unipolar patients, respectively. Gershon and co-workers (1982)
have suggested a continuum of severity with the nonpsychotic
unipolar patients being least severe and the psychotic or
"schizoaffective" bipolar patients being the most severe. These
authors found a decreasing lifetime prevalence for major affective disorders in the relatives of the various groups with a systematic decrease from schizoaffective through nonpsychotic
unipolar to normality. We tested the hypothesis in the separated groups of bipolar/nonpsychotic, bipolar/psychotic,
unipolar/nonpsychotic, and unipolar/psychotic. The data are
shown in Table 8–3. There was no difference between the bipo-
lar/nonpsychotic and the bipolar/psychotic groups nor was
there any difference between the unipolar groups. What is most
interesting is that the bipolar/psychotic, presumably the most
severe group, has a slightly lower occurrence of familial affec-

**Table 8–3.**  Familial affective disorder of bipolar and unipolar
probands, separated according to psychosis

|  | Parents and siblings at risk | Ill | Morbid risk (%) |
|---|---|---|---|
| Bipolar nonpsychotic | 139 | 18 | 13 |
| Bipolar psychotic | 267 | 35 | 13 |
| Unipolar nonpsychotic | 340 | 51 | 15 |
| Unipolar psychotic | 459 | 70 | 15 |

*Source.*  Adapted from Winokur 1984.

tive disorder than the unipolar/nonpsychotic. These data support the argument that there is no continuum of severity that would manifest itself in a larger family history the closer one gets to the top of the group on severity (i.e., the bipolar/psychotic).

## Linkage in Bipolar Illness

In a clinical genetic study of X linkage in bipolar illness, the presence of such a type of transmission would be related to more females being ill in the population. Ill mothers should have an equal number of ill sons and daughters, assuming the penetrance factors were the same in both sexes, and there should be an absence of ill-father/ill-son groupings. In a sense, the hallmark of X-linked dominant transmission is the lack of ill-father/ill-son transmissions. Such findings were reported by Winokur (1970) in a study with 17 ill-mother/ill-son pairs but no ill-father/ill-son pairs. In the Iowa 500 study, we made an effort to look at this type of transmission. In the 109 patients who were either bipolar at admission or became bipolar in the short-term chart follow-up, 58% of the probands were female. The expectation in X-linked dominant transmission, assuming that only one kind of transmission was present for an illness, would be higher. At least two-thirds of the manic-depressive patients should be female. Further studying of the parental matings in the male patients showed 4% of the fathers and 10% of the mothers suffered an affective disorder. For female patients, 11% of the fathers and 5% of the mothers were similarly affected. Thus, though there is an excess of mothers transmitting the illness to the male patients, it is clear that X-linked transmission could not be the only type of transmission because if X linkage were the sole means of transmission no fathers could transmit the illness to their sons.

In the bipolar patients, other transmission possibilities were entertained. The patients were separated into an early and late onset group. Early onset was related to onset occurring at an age younger than 30, and late onset related to an age older than 30. In the early onset patients, 5% of the fathers were ill with affective disorder, and in the late onset patients, 14% of the fathers were ill. Affectively ill mothers in the early onset group were at 8% and at 5% for the late onset group. In the early onset probands, 7% of the siblings were ill with affective disorder as compared with 6% in the late onset patients. None of these differences are significant. There was no evidence that the late onset is associated with a lesser genetic background (Winokur 1975b).

## Familial Distinction of Hebephrenic and Paranoid Schizophrenia

Using the original clinical diagnoses of hebephrenic and paranoid schizophrenia, we assessed family differences (Winokur et al. 1974). Some findings from the literature suggested that hebephrenic patients have an increased family history of schizophrenia over paranoid patients. Also, other data suggest that the schizophrenia subtype breeds true in that hebephrenic patients are more likely to have hebephrenic relatives, and paranoid patients are more likely to have paranoid relatives. This latter finding would suggest that paranoid schizophrenia and hebephrenic schizophrenia are two distinct kinds of diseases (Böök 1953; Kallman 1938; Schulz 1932). Clinically, in the Iowa 500 sample, the two groups differed in that hebephrenic patients have more abnormal affect, more tangential thinking, block more, and are more incoherent. Paranoid schizophrenic patients were admitted at an older age, were older at onset, and showed less of a disruption of family life. The blind family history assessment revealed that hebephrenic probands had three times as many schizophrenic relatives as the paranoid probands. These differences between the two groups support the possibility that process or chronic schizophrenia might not be a unitary or a homogeneous illness and that there are two types of schizophrenia, one of which might manifest itself mostly as hebephrenia but occasionally as paranoid schizophrenia. The second type would be paranoid schizophrenia in which there is a paucity of schizophrenic relatives. In fact, this finding may be flawed by the fact that the Feighner criteria pick up patients with delusional disorder as paranoid schizophrenic, and there were some patients in the study who were diagnosed as having paranoia (delusional disorder). It is possible that the familial differences that were found (although not significant) might have reflected an admixture of schizophrenic and delusional disorder patients where the delusional disorder group might have a different kind of family history (Winokur 1985). Also, no data existed in the study to suggest breeding true (i.e., that hebephrenic patients had hebephrenic relatives and paranoid patients had paranoid relatives), which would be an absolute necessity for a two-illness concept in schizophrenia. Thus, though 2.4% of the relatives of hebephrenic patients had schizophrenia as opposed to only .8% of the paranoid patients' relatives, there are a variety of possible explanations that do not support the concept of two types of schizophrenia. In order to support this concept more strongly, subsequent data using follow-up material enabled us to look at this more directly.

## Family History and Good Outcome and Poor Outcome Schizophrenia

To assess family history and its relationship to recovery, the 315 excluded clinically diagnosed schizophrenic patients were evaluated and compared to the Iowa 500 (Winokur and Tsuang 1975a). Of these, 63 patients had at some point made a complete recovery, and 144 had never been well since index admission. One hundred and eight of the 315 cases were classified uncertain as to recovery and were not evaluated. Sixty-three recovered patients were compared with the 144 nonrecovered patients on a number of variables. For the recovered patients, there was a significant increase in the diagnosis of catatonic schizophrenia: 21% versus 10% ($P$ = .05). One of the findings was that recovered schizophrenic patients were more likely to come from families where two or more family members had been ill with a clearly remitting illness. Such a clustering of remitting illnesses would be an unlikely finding in the nonrecovered schizophrenic patients' families. If one evaluated the Iowa 500 patients who did meet the Feighner criteria for schizophrenia and divided them into 15 recovered and 114 nonrecovered, there was no increase in remitting illnesses in the families of the small number of recovered patients. There was an increase or a trend for more paranoid schizophrenic patients to be found in the recovered group. Again, it is conceivable that some of these people who were considered recovered, in fact, did not have paranoid schizophrenia but may have had delusional disorder. Thus, the use of strict Feighner criteria for the diagnosis of schizophrenia is predictive of a bad prognosis, and when one looks at those few patients who did improve, no significant family differences were found. However, in patients who did not meet strict criteria, the family history of remitting illness in more than one family member might be helpful in suggesting a better outcome.

In general, it is clear that the blind family history supported the differentiation between schizophrenia and the affective disorders. It was useful in separating subtypes of unipolar depression; however, it showed no difference between psychotic and nonpsychotic affective disorders. It was not very useful separating subtypes of schizophrenia although there were some hints in the data that the schizophrenic patient with a good prognosis might be related to a family history of remitting illness, particularly if the schizophrenic patient did not meet full research criteria. There was no evidence in favor of X linkage in bipolar illness in this analysis. The data did support the probability that there were two types of unipolar depression, one associated with familial alcoholism (depression spectrum disease) and the other not (pure depressive disease). Thus, the family history method used in this workup contributed in defining specific illnesses in the Iowa 500 patients.

# Chapter 9

# Special Aspects

*Life Events, Parental Loss, Premorbid
Asociality, Clinical Characteristics,
Outcome, Bipolar Heterogeneity, Subtyping
Schizophrenia, Delusional Disorder,
Affective Symptoms in Schizophrenia,
Sporadic Depressive Disease*

As in any large and complex data set that contains many variables, it was possible to use the Iowa 500 study to investigate a number of important questions. Interestingly, the data were not collected with the eye to looking at these special aspects, which makes such analyses more reliable in that they were not subject to any halo effect. In the data collection, no specific effort was being made to prove any points on these questions, and, consequently, one might be inclined to place some confidence in the findings. On the other hand, it should be noted that research hypotheses were not formulated to test some of these interesting questions. Each succeeding section stands independently, as each is the product of special interests on the part of separate investigators.

The question might arise as to why each of these small projects was done. The answer is simple enough. These projects were reflections of specific interests on the part of the investigators. In some cases, the material was gleaned from the original assessments of the chart material (see Appendix II). In other cases, the investigators went back to the original charts in order to obtain more information. There was considerable confidence in the research diagnoses that were made of these patients. As a consequence, the investigators noted the accessibility of well-diagnosed patients and looked for specific clinical and etiologic associations. The diagnoses were very reliable for such things as a major depression, a bipolar illness, or a clear and unequivocal schizophrenic illness. This allowed us to use these patients to determine such things as heterogeneity within the large category of schizophrenia or the presence of psychosocial factors associated with each of the major diagnoses. Interestingly, even now these data could be used for further research into questions related to the major psychoses.

━━━━━━━━━━━━━━━━━━━━━━━━━━━━━━━━━━━━━━━━

## Life Events in Schizophrenia and the Primary Affective Disorders

At the time of patient selection and diagnosis, the presence of adverse life events as noted by the psychiatrists and social workers was recorded. Significant precipitating events were found in a minority of the three diagnostic groups (Clancy et al. 1973), although some differences did exist. The presence of any precipitant was found in 39% of the unipolar depressive and 27% of the bipolar depressive but in only 11% of the schizophrenic patients. By chi-square analysis, this distribution shows a significant difference ($P = .001$) with the schizophrenic patients showing fewer precipitating events. For the unipolar, bipolar, and schizophrenic patients, psychological precipitants were seen in 17%, 9%, and 4%, respectively ($P = .001$); for physical precipitants, 5%, 12%, and 3% ($P = .01$), respectively; and for social precipitants 5%, 0%, and 1% ($P = .01$), respectively. The unipolar patients showed 5% who were considered to have menopausal precipitants as opposed to none of the bipolar and .5% the schizophrenic patients ($P = .01$). This is probably simply a reflection of the older age of the unipolar depressive patients at onset and also at time of admission. Postpartum precipitants were seen in 3.5% of the unipolar, 6% of the bipolar, and 2.5% of the schizophrenic patients. This was a nonsignificant difference. The overall results support a trend for significant life events to be encountered most frequently in the unipolar depressive patients and least frequently in the schizophrenic patients with the bipolar patients falling in between. Depression seems to be the most likely syndrome associated with life events of all of the illnesses that we studied. This finding fits in well with the concept of reactive or situationally precipitated depression.

The findings are especially of interest because in this study we were dealing with the pure sample composed of patients with primary affective disorder or schizophrenia. Excluded from the sample were patients with symptoms that could be attributed to some other kind of psychiatric disease or physical illness (secondary syndromes). In the case of secondary syndromes, particularly secondary depression, it would be far easier to find precipitating factors. Indeed, the primary illness itself (i.e., the medical disease or the psychiatric disease) could be considered a precipitating factor.

## The Association Between Early Parental Loss and Diagnosis

The frequency of parental loss and parental death among 129 depressive, 155 schizophrenic, and 63 manic patients from the Iowa 500 data set was investigated (Pfohl et al. 1983). These data were recorded at the time of the original assessment of the charts of the patients. The number of patients with specific diagnoses that were investigated is lower than the number that entered the study because the research methodology included a logistic regression to control for such confounders as social class, sibship size, parental age at birth, and patient's age at admission. As not all patients had complete data on these confounders, only the index cases that contained data on all this material were used, the others being eliminated from the statistical workup. Depressive patients were found to experience early maternal death (prior to age 18) 3.4 times more frequently than schizophrenic patients and 2.1 times more frequently than the bipolar patients. There is no comparison with control subjects. In the logistic regression, diagnosis was the dependent variable, and the regression model included the patient's sex, age at admission, maternal age at patient's birth, family rank, and father's occupation. When these variables were controlled, there was a significant increase in maternal death among depressive over schizophrenic patients. But in the other comparisons, depressive versus manic the patients and schizophrenic patients versus manic patients, the differences were not significant. There was no significant finding with regard to maternal separation, only maternal death. Regarding paternal death, there was no significant finding between the three diagnostic groups. Paternal death did not separate the three groups but paternal separation was 3.1% in the depressive patients, 12.9% in the schizophrenic patients, and 4.8% in manic patients. However, when the confounders were taken into account in the logistic regression, this finding washed out and was not significant. Most of the findings regarding paternal separations were explained by divorce among the parents of the schizophrenic patients. Thus, the major finding in this study was that maternal death was more frequently associated with the diagnosis of depression. Importantly, of the 16 cases of maternal death before proband age of 18, only one was attributable to suicide. There is some support for the hypothesis that the experience of early maternal death might be relatively more important as a risk factor for depression than for schizophrenia, but the rather low frequency of maternal death suggests that the issue is of more theoretical than practical clinical importance.

## Schizophrenia With Premorbid Asociality

In an effort to test whether there might be heterogeneity in schizophrenia, the Iowa 500 schizophrenic patients and the discarded clinically diagnosed schizophrenic patients were divided into those who had premorbid asociality and those who did not show this kind of personality (Quitkin et al. 1980). Premorbid asociality is the term that is used when the schizophrenic patient shows social incompetence in the context of being friendless and scapegoated during childhood, with academic difficulty and a limited set of interests. Premorbid asociality was assessed from the psychiatric and social work notes in the charts. The family history of schizophrenia was investigated between the premorbidly asocial and nonpremorbidly asocial schizophrenic patients. The proportion of families of premorbidly asocial schizophrenic patients ($n = 24$) with schizophrenia in relatives was 0%. Of 476 nonpremorbidly asocial schizophrenic patients, 34 (7.1%) had a family history of schizophrenia. The difference is not significant but is consistent with the possibility that subtle forms of central nervous system damage occurring early may result in neurologic soft signs and premorbid asociality. Against this hypothesis is the idea that hebephrenic-catatonic schizophrenia is usually associated with more premorbid asociality than paranoid schizophrenia and also possibly a larger family history of schizophrenia (Winokur et al. 1974).

## Clinical Characteristics

Some of the clinical characteristics are given in Table 9–1. Of course, the differences between schizophrenic, manic, and depressive patients are to be expected with those symptoms that were used for making diagnoses; however, it is interesting to note the differences in percentages among the various groups.

Paranoid and hebephrenic schizophrenic patients were also compared. In this case, the diagnosis that was used is essentially the diagnosis made by the clinicians at the Iowa Psychopathic Hospital. These differences are shown in Table 9–2, where one finding of interest is the fact that the hebephrenic patients show a large number of probands with motor symptoms (36%). The association of hebephrenic symptoms with catatonic symptoms in the chronic schizophrenic patients is also characteristic of the patients in the study by Böök (1953). The follow-up status of paranoid schizophrenic patients is strikingly better than that in the hebephrenic schizophrenic patients. As noted before, however, paranoid schizophrenic patients probably contained an admixture of delusional disorder patients in that such

**Table 9–1.**    Clinical characteristics of schizophrenic, manic, and depressive patients

|  | Schizophrenic (*n* = 200) | Bipolar[a] (*n* = 100[a]) | Depressive (*n* = 225) |
|---|---|---|---|
| Age at onset, median years | 26 | 27 | 39 |
| Weight loss, % | 7 | 12 | 39 |
| Energy loss, % | 23 | 11 | 70 |
| Terminal insomnia, % | 2 | 12 | 18 |
| Euphoric or irritable, % | 2 | 94 | 0 |
| Extravagance, % | 2 | 19 | 0 |
| Social withdrawal, % | 72 | 3 | 32 |
| Primary delusions, % | 25 | 4 | 4 |
| Persecutory delusions, % | 42 | 25 | 17 |
| Auditory hallucinations, % | 54 | 15 | 6 |
| Haptic hallucinations, % | 29 | 5 | 8 |
| Motor symptoms (tics, stereotypies, verbigerations, grimacing, waxy flexibility, posturing), % | 32 | 11 | 2 |

[a]94 manic and 6 bipolar depressive patients.
*Source.*   Adapted from Winokur 1975a.

**Table 9–2.** Comparison of paranoid and hebephrenic
schizophrenic patients

| Symptoms | Hebephrenic (%) | Paranoid (%) |
|---|---|---|
| Symbolism | 20 | 41 |
| Tangentiality | 57 | 20 |
| Motor symptoms | 36 | 12 |
| Inappropriate affect | 19 | 6 |
| Follow-up (2–10+ years) complete recovery | 9 | 30 |
| Held a job after index admit | 23 | 70 |
| Family history, proportion of schizophrenic relatives | 2.4 | 0.8 |

*Note.* Percentages based on varying numbers of hebephrenic and paranoid
schizophrenic patients because of lost information in follow-up.
*Source.* Adapted from Winokur 1975a.

patients meet the Feighner criteria for schizophrenia. This
would affect the results since it is possible that delusional disorder patients have a better prognosis than schizophrenic patients. Blocking was three times as frequent in hebephrenic
than in paranoid patients, but primary delusions were twice as
frequent in the paranoid patients as were haptic hallucinations.
Auditory and visual hallucinations were not markedly different,
though 31% of the hebephrenic patients had visual hallucinations as opposed to 21% of the paranoid patients.

## Elation Versus Irritability in Mania

In the Feighner research criteria, irritability is given equal
status with elation as a mood state for the diagnosis of mania.
Winokur and Tsuang (1975b) evaluated 96 of the 100 bipolar

patients who were manic at index admission. Of these, 8 were considered irritable only in mood, 28 euphoric only, and 58 euphoric and irritable. The 8 patients who showed no elation were compared with the 86 who showed euphoria or euphoria and irritability, and we found some clinical differences. Irritable manic patients tended to be less grandiose and less frequently showed the symptom of increased money spending (extravagance) and were less likely to show flight of ideas. There was little difference in follow-up with 63% of the irritable only patients having a complete recovery at some point in follow-up as compared with 44% of those who were elated or elated and irritable. A cluster of symptoms seems to be associated with euphoria, including flight of ideas; grandiosity, which may or may not be delusional; and increased spending. These symptoms are all less frequent in the patients who showed only irritability.

## Organic and Psychotic Symptoms in the Affective Disorders

Psychotic symptoms (delusions and hallucinations) as well as symptoms of an abnormal sensorium were evaluated in unipolar versus bipolar depressive patients. Sixty percent of bipolar depressive patients had psychotic symptoms as opposed to 57% of the unipolar depressive patients. There was also no significant difference in the two groups as regards sensorium defects. Interestingly, 21% of manic patients had auditory hallucinations versus only 6% of bipolar depressive patients (Kathol and Winokur 1977).

Regarding all bipolar (mainly manic at index admission) versus unipolar depressive patients, there is no significant difference between the two groups in passivity delusions, depersonalization or derealization, altered perception, symbolism, or persecutory delusions and/or thought broadcasting and/or other delusions. However, auditory hallucinations are more frequent in the bipolar patients as are visual hallucinations and motor symptoms. There is no difference of any significance between haptic hallucinations and disorientation during index admission (Winokur 1984).

We found the course of the illness to be similar in psychotic versus nonpsychotic affective disorder patients. In a comparison of 59 nonpsychotic bipolar and 54 psychotic bipolar patients who were approximately the same age at index and were followed through essentially the same amount of time, those who were psychotic were significantly more likely to be first-admission patients. However, there was no difference between psychotic and nonpsychotic bipolar patients on improvement at discharge, continuous hospitalization in short-term follow-up, or complete recovery during follow-up. In a comparison of nonpsychotic and psychotic unipolar patients who were the same age at index, the psychotic patients were more likely to be first-episode patients, less likely to be markedly improved at index discharge, and less likely to make a complete recovery during follow-up. However, the follow-up in the nonpsychotic patients was 57 months versus only 35 months for the psychotic patients, and it is therefore possible that the extra time for the nonpsychotic patients to get well accounts for this difference (Winokur 1984).

## Aspects of Outcome After a Short Follow-Up

In a short follow-up (1 or more years), which was accomplished by reviewing the notations made by the social workers and physicians in the patient's chart, we found that diagnostic stability over time was quite good. From the data given in Table 9–3, it is notable that 98%–99% of schizophrenic patients do not change their diagnosis, 76%–88% of bipolar patients do not change their diagnosis, and 88%–94% of unipolar depressive patients do not change their diagnosis. Follow-up diagnoses were made by different clinicians than those who made the original index diagnoses or the research diagnoses. The results suggest considerable validity in the use of rigorous diagnostic criteria (Winokur 1974a). Of some importance is the fact that of the 11 patients who went from affective disorder to schizophrenia in the short follow-up, 6 were diagnosed as having catatonic schizophrenia—a diagnosis that carries with it more remissions and a different family history from other types of schizophrenia.

Clinical and course differences related to sex, age at onset, and age at index in unipolar depressive patients were assessed by comparing the original 101 unipolar depressive males with 124 unipolar depressive females. Females were noted to be sig-

**Table 9–3.**　Changes in diagnosis of schizophrenia, mania, and depression after follow-up of 1 or more years

| | Diagnosing with use of "research criteria" | | |
|---|---|---|---|
| | S | B | D |
| Number at index admission | 200 | 100 | 225 |
| Patients followed for 1 or more years | 151 (76%) | 66 (66%) | 171 (76%) |
| Mean follow-up period, years | 3 | 3 | 5 |
| Follow-up clinical diagnosis: | | | |
| 　No further diagnosis | 65 | 33 | 96 |
| 　Depressive illness | 0 | 6 | 56 |
| 　Manic-depressive illness | 0 | 19 | 10 |
| 　Schizophrenia | 84 | 6 | 5 |
| 　Other | 2 | 2 | 4 |
| Unchanged from schizophrenia or affective disorder in those having subsequent diagnosis, % | 98 | 76 | 88 |
| Unchanged from schizophrenia or affective disorder, % | 99 | 88 | 94 |

*Note.*　S = schizophrenic; B = bipolar; D = depressive.
*Source.*　Adapted from Winokur 1974a.

nificantly more likely to have agitation and precipitating factors than males. Males, though, were more likely to have psychomotor retardation (79% versus 52%; $P = .0005$). When comparing early onset (before 40) to late onset (after 40) unipolar depressive patients, the early onset patients were more likely to be discharged to the community (i.e., less likely to be chronic, less likely to be agitated, more likely to be retarded, and more likely to show diurnal variation). All of these differences were significant. When patients were compared on the basis of being young (index age under 40) and old (index age over 40) at time of index admission, the young patients were less likely to be agitated, more likely to be retarded, and less likely to be ill 6 months or more at index admission (Winokur et al. 1973). Chronicity in females increased with age and seemed to be more related to index age than age at onset, whereas further episodes occurred more frequently in males and seemed to be related to age at index rather than in age at onset (Winokur 1974b). Notably, the differences in course were probably more related to age at index than to age at onset in this data set. Of course, age at admission is a more reliable measurement than age at onset of illness, which always requires some judgment. These two measurements are highly correlated, however.

## Heterogeneity and Course in Bipolar Illness

Though bipolar illness appears quite homogeneous, it is entirely possible that there is more than one autonomous illness within that diagnosis. There are findings in other studies that indicate that some, but not all, bipolar patients show X-linked genetic transmission in their families (Winokur et al. 1969). This kind of heterogeneity, such as the observation that a subset of bipolar patients may show X linkage, would suggest that perhaps other kinds of heterogeneity exist also, such as bipolar patients who have abnormal electroencephalograms (EEGs) and who are less likely to have a positive family history of bipolar illness than those with normal EEGs (Kadrmas and Winokur 1979). It seemed that various other possibilities might exist for determining heterogeneity and course in manic-depressive illness (Winokur 1975b). Separating 109 bipolar patients by sex, 63% of the female bipolar patients had an onset prior to age 30 as opposed to 37% of the males. For late onset patients, however, there was no difference, with 50% of those that had an onset over 30 being male and 50% being female. These differences, though suggestive, are not significant. It does seem possible that females may be more likely to have an early onset but this is not proven. However, prior to index hospitalization, females were more likely to have had more episodes and more previous hospitalizations than males even though they were exactly the same age at admission, which suggests that there may be something clinically significant in an earlier onset for females. Also in the short follow-up, 42% of females had a subsequent episode as opposed to 57% of males. There were, however, almost twice as many subsequent hospitalizations per person among males when compared with females. These data suggest that females have more episodes early and males have more episodes later on, but the data are not definitive.

Median age at onset among bipolar patients was 30, and a comparison of early and late onset patients showed no significant differences or trends in course, either before or after index hospitalization. In this particular sample, neither sex nor age at onset seemed related to family history of any particular type. There was an interesting finding, however. If one compared bipolar patients with one or more prior episodes to those patients who entered for first episode, there was a significant difference in follow-up. Table 9–4 shows that first-episode patients were much more likely to have a subsequent episode (91% versus 53%; $P = .05$). This finding suggests the possibility that as a group, bipolar patients are likely to suffer from a flurry of episodes, which will then die down in the course of time. These data are also in keeping with a report by Saran (1969) that bipolar patients were more likely to have a further remission in the immediate follow-up period of 2 years than they were in a subsequent 2-year period after the first 2 years had passed. If bipolar illness does manifest itself by clusters of episodes and then becomes relatively quiescent, this has significant meaning about interpreting improvement with treatment modalities that are used for prophylaxis.

## The Criteria for Subtyping Schizophrenia

By use of Feighner criteria, it was possible to obtain a group of 200 "process" schizophrenic patients that was unique for studies performed in the early 1970s. For these patients, there were subtype diagnoses made between 1934 and 1944 by staff psychiatrists. But how meaningful these subtype diagnoses might be and whether they contribute anything to the understanding of chronic schizophrenia were important questions to be asked. In an attempt to answer these questions, Tsuang and Winokur (1974) evaluated the difference between hebephrenic and paranoid schizophrenic patients as diagnosed by the clinicians between 1934 and 1944. Table 9–5 shows some of the clinical differences between the hebephrenic and paranoid patients.

**Table 9–4.**   Follow-up (2–20 years) of manic probands according to prior history

|  | Patients with one or more episodes | First-episode patients |
|---|---|---|
| Number of patients | 19 | 11 |
| Mean follow-up, years | 5.6 | 5.1 |
| Episodes per person | 1.1 | 1.4 |
| Proportion with subsequent episode in follow-up | 53% | 91% |

*Source.*   Adapted from Winokur 1975b.

These included more blocking, formal thought disorder, and inappropriate affect in the former. All of these patients were younger than 40 years of age at index admission. This group was chosen in order to control for the possible effect of age on symptomatology. Of course, some of these findings are expected in that the symptoms were part of the diagnostic criteria used at that time. One unexpected finding was a clear indication of memory deficit being more frequent among hebephrenic rather than paranoid patients.

Hebephrenic patients were far less likely to have a good prognosis for recovery or productive work in the follow-up (Table 9–2). Table 9–6 presents some other clear differences between the hebephrenic and paranoid schizophrenic patients. As motor symptoms were so frequent in the hebephrenic patients, the more appropriate term would be hebephrenic-catatonic schizophrenia. On the basis of these findings and a discriminate

**Table 9–5.**    Symptom differences between hebephrenic-catatonic and paranoid patients

| | Hebephrenic $N = 112$ n (%) | Paranoid $N = 49$ n (%) |
|---|---|---|
| Median age at index admission | 25 | 31 |
| Index admission, first admission | 88 (79) | 31 (76) |
| Symbolism (primary delusions)[*] | 22 (20) | 20 (41) |
| Blocking[**] | 32 (29 | 6 (12) |
| Tangentiality[***] | 64 (57) | 10 (20) |
| Motor symptoms[*] | 40 (36) | 6 (12) |
| Inappropriate affect[**] | 21 (19) | 3 (6) |
| Memory deficit[*] | 16 (14) | 1 (2) |

[*]$P < .05;$ [**]$P < .01;$ [***]$P < .001.$
*Source.*    Adapted from Tsuang and Winokur 1974.

**Table 9–6.** Hebephrenic-catatonic versus paranoid schizophrenic patients

| Clinical features | Hebephrenic | Paranoid |
|---|---|---|
| Age at onset before 25 | Likely | Less likely |
| Marriage | Less likely | More likely |
| Employment | Less likely | More likely |
| Family history of schizophrenia | More likely | Less likely |
| Disorganized thought: tangential, illogical, incoherent, or irrelevant speech; loose associations, blocking, or other formal thought disorders | + + | + or − |
| Affect changes: inappropriate affect, giggling, self-absorbed, smiling, mood inconsistent with expressed ideas | + + | + or − |
| Flat affect, frozen, expressionless, impenetrable face | + + | + or − |
| Behavior symptoms: bizarre behavior, unpredictable, inappropriate, unusual, irresponsible, purposeless, or withdrawn behavior not in keeping with socio-cultural norms | + + | + or − |
| Motor symptoms, hebephrenic traits— habitual mannerisms of an ordinary character, usually involving a single part of the body (e.g., tics, grimaces, moving lips soundlessly, fidgeting with fingers, hand wringing, thigh rubbing) | + + | + or − |
| Catatonic traits—physical activity of an extraordinary and abnormal character, usually involving the whole body (e.g., posturing, stereotyping, waxy flexibility, negativism, stupor, hyperkinesis) | + | − |
| Delusions or hallucinations, persecution, passivity, control, symbolism (primary delusions), thought broadcasting, experiences or alienation, complete auditory hallucinations, delusional perceptions, or hallucinations in any sensory modality | + or − | + + |

*Note.* Traits present to a marked degree or of a persistent nature (+ +); present to a mild degree or of a transient nature (+); absent (−).
*Source.* Adapted from Tsuang and Winokur 1974.

function analysis that showed that age at onset, disorganized thoughts, and affect changes were the best subset of three variables in distinguishing paranoid from nonparanoid schizophrenia, we came up with a set of criteria for hebephrenic-catatonic schizophrenia. After having made a Feighner criteria diagnosis of schizophrenia, patients could now be differentiated into those with hebephrenic-catatonic schizophrenia (nonparanoid) and paranoid schizophrenia. If the criteria were not met, then the diagnoses of chronic undifferentiated schizophrenia or schizophrenia, subtype undermined, might be used.

---

## Hebephrenic-Catatonic Versus Paranoid Schizophrenia

I. Hebephrenic-catatonic (A through D must be present)
   A. One of the following:
      1. Age at onset under 25 years
      2. Unmarried or unemployed
      3. Family history of schizophrenia
   B. Disorganized thought
   C. Affect changes (1 or 2)
      1. Inappropriate affect
      2. Flat affect
   D. Behavioral symptoms (1 or 2)
      1. Bizarre behavior
      2. Motor symptoms (a or b)
         a. Hebephrenic traits
         b. Catatonic traits (if present, subtype may be modified to hebephrenia with catatonic traits)
II. Paranoid (A through C must be present)
   A. One of the following:
      1. Age at onset after 25 years
      2. Married or employed
      3. Absence of family history of schizophrenia
   B. Exclusion criteria

    1. Disorganized thoughts must be absent or of mild degree such that speech is intelligible

    2. Affective and behavioral symptoms, as described in hebephrenia, must be absent or of mild degree

C. Preoccupation with extensive, well-organized delusions or hallucinations

Types I and II may be utilized independently to classify process schizophrenia into either paranoid/nonparanoid or hebephrenic/nonhebephrenic types, depending on the requirements of individual researchers. We, however, attempted to formulate criteria because our studies had indicated to us that subtype differentiation can be supported by the available data, and that such differentiation has predictive value for the course and outcome of the patient and might be relevant to the prediction of familial risk for schizophrenia. Since such criteria may lead to the ability to select homogeneous illnesses, the need for such converging data is clear. With such pure subgroups to work with, it would be possible to determine biological or psychosocial causes that might otherwise cancel each other out. Regarding research criteria that we actually developed, we do not contend that their degrees of inclusiveness and exclusiveness are perfect at this stage. Such a determination awaits the results of clinical experience and further research, employing these criteria, in order that data from various centers can be compared and validated.

The criteria are presented with the idea that they may be used to evaluate subsequent data on course, etiology, treatment, and family background of schizophrenic patients who present with clinical syndromes that are different, with the purpose of possibly identifying different illnesses. An early test of the hypothesis that these might be useful was presented by Winokur and Tsuang (1981). Twenty-nine patients of the Iowa 500 who were originally diagnosed as having paranoid schizophrenia and in follow-up continued to have that diagnosis using the Tsuang/Winokur criteria were matched with 29 patients who had nonparanoid schizophrenia (hebephrenic-catatonic). Though there was an attempt made to match the patients on the basis of sex, age, and marital status, this proved impossible. The paranoid schizophrenic patients were older than the 29 nonparanoid schizophrenic patients ($P = .005$), where the paranoid patients were 37 at admission and the nonparanoid patients were 31. In fact, 34% of the paranoid schizophrenic patients were older than 40 at admission. None of the nonparanoid schizophrenic patients were older than 40 at admission. However, for this study, the analysis was controlled for sex. Also, there was no obvious difference in ages of mothers at birth of proband, and between 26% and 28% of both groups were born in the winter months of December, January, and February.

There was a rather complete set of data on blood and spinal fluid findings in these patients because in the early days at the Iowa Psychopathic Hospital almost all patients received a lumbar puncture. The spinal fluid protein did not differentiate the two groups, and the white cell count was essentially the same. However, there was a difference in percent of lymphocytes. The mean for both groups was 24.4% of lymphocytes in the white blood cell count. Paranoid schizophrenic patients were below the mean in 48%, which would be expected, but the nonparanoid schizophrenic patients were below the mean in 76%. This was a significant difference at the .05 level of probability. The difference in lymphocyte count is totally unexplained but would be in keeping with the possibility that paranoid and hebephrenic schizophrenia differ in severity or that they may have different etiologies. Likewise, these patients were compared by family history of schizophrenia where the morbid risk for schizophrenia was 7.7% for paranoid patients, and for 29 nonparanoid patients it was 12.9%. This difference is not significant, but it is interesting that there is a 67% increase in the family members of the nonparanoid schizophrenic patients. Of 49 interviewed relatives of the 29 paranoid schizophrenic patients, 3 were schizophrenic, but of the nonparanoid schizophrenic patients of 56 relatives, 6 were schizophrenic. Though this may not reflect any important difference, it does suggest that it might be worthwhile to look at larger samples.

## The Emergence of Delusional Disorder (Paranoia) From the Schizophrenic Patients of the Iowa 500

As mentioned previously, the criteria that were used to identify the schizophrenic patients in the Iowa 500 were such that they would have also included any patient with a chronic nonaffective, nonorganic psychosis. This means that the criteria would have picked up patients who had delusional disorder because these patients are generally chronic, do not suffer from major affective episodes, and share some symptoms with schizophrenic patients, namely delusions. These delusions are generally quite implausible but not impossible. A description of simple delusional disorder has been presented by Winokur (1977). As defined, simple delusional disorder may contain implausible delusions but few, if any, other kinds of schizophrenia-type symptoms. There is a group that shares aspects of both paranoid schizophrenia and simple delusional disorder that might be called hallucinatory delusional disorder. This would describe an individual who has chronic implausible delusions but also has hallucinations. The appropriate role of hallucinatory delusional disorder in terms of its relationship to either simple delusional disorder or schizophrenia has not been finally decided. A classification of the chronic psychoses would include simple delusional disorder, hallucinatory delusional disorder, paranoid schizophrenia, and hebephrenic-catatonic schizophrenia (Winokur 1986). How many of the 200 Feighner schizophrenic patients might have had delusional disorder is unknown, but it may be possible to obtain a rough estimate.

Of the 200 schizophrenic patients, 29 were originally diagnosed as having paranoid schizophrenia by the Feighner criteria at time of entry into this study and continued to have that diagnosis at follow-up 30–40 years later. We did not have the clinical information at the time of the follow-up. But certainly at the time of admission we were able to decide whether any of those 29 paranoid schizophrenic patients might have met the criteria for simple delusional disorder, and we found that 10 of the 29, in fact, did meet these criteria. Of course, it is entirely possible that of the 200 original schizophrenic patients of the Iowa 500 a few more might have met the criteria, but that would have to be evaluated separately. What was particularly interesting was that of the 10 patients who met the criteria for simple delusional disorder at the time of admission 2 had family members with traits of suspiciousness, jealousy, secretiveness, paranoid behavior, and delusions. These were the symptoms and personality traits that were seen in a prior study of patients with delusional disorder (Winokur 1985). None of the 19 remaining paranoid schizophrenic patients had such traits in family members. The amount of imprecision in the diagnosis of the original 200 schizophrenic patients is impossible to assess at this point. Certainly, 10 of 200 suggests that at least 5% might have delusional disorder, but it may be more. The impurity that is contributed by the delusional disorder patients is of some importance because if, in fact, delusional disorder patients have a different prognosis than schizophrenic patients, the studies of the course of schizophrenia might also be somewhat imperfect. It is, therefore, quite possible that, when dealing with chronic nonaffective psychoses, we are dealing with two sets of spectra. One is a schizophrenia spectrum, which includes schizophrenia, schizotypal personality, and schizoid personality; the other is the paranoia spectrum (or delusional disorder spectrum), which includes delusional disorder, paranoid personalities, and such traits as secretiveness, jealousy, and suspiciousness.

## The Role of Affective Symptoms in Rigorously Diagnosed Schizophrenia

Affective type symptomatology seems to be rather ubiquitous, as shown in Figure 9–1, which presents the presence of depressive and manic symptoms in the 200 schizophrenic patients. The modal number of depressive symptoms is three and the

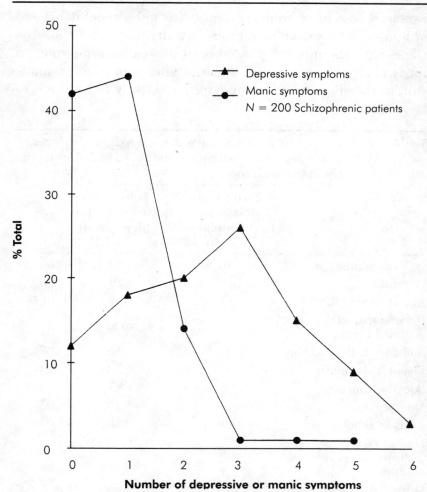

**Figure 9–1.**   Presence of depressive and manic symptoms in the 200 schizophrenic patients at admission.

modal number of manic symptoms is one; thus, almost an equal number of schizophrenic patients have no manic symptoms. If one separates those schizophrenic patients with the presence or absence of the depressive symptoms that are seen in the Feighner criteria, Table 9–7 shows some of the differences between those schizophrenic patients with and without depressive symptoms. Of particular interest are the facts that those patients with the minimum number of depressive symptoms are more likely to be continuously hospitalized since index admission in the short follow-up and are more likely to have schizo-

**Table 9–7.** Differences between schizophrenic patients with zero to one depressive symptoms and those with four to six depressive symptoms

| | Zero to one symptoms (%) (not depressed) N = 50 | Four to six symptoms (%) (depressed) N = 52[a] | P |
|---|---|---|---|
| < 30 at admission | 46 | 81 | .0005 |
| Paranoid | 44 | 19 | .002 |
| Age at onset < 19 | 12 | 37 | .005 |
| Depersonalization, derealization | 8 | 25 | .01 |
| Auditory hallucinations | 46 | 65 | .07 |
| Visual hallucinations | 14 | 33 | .04 |
| Social withdrawal | 50 | 83 | .0005 |
| Memory deficit | 4 | 19 | .03 |
| Antisocial behavior | 16 | 4 | .04 |
| Morbid risk, affective disorder, parents, and siblings | 3 | 6 | NS |
| Morbid risk, schizophrenia, parents, and siblings | 3 | 1 | NS |
| Affective disorder in extended family | 6 | 13 | NS |
| Schizophrenia in extended family | 7 | 1 | .05 |
| Continuous hospitalization since index | 46 | 23 | .025 |
| Subsequent episodes | 10 | 18 | NS |

*Note.* NS = not significant.
[a]98 patients had between two and three depressive symptoms.

phrenia in an extended family member. There are also some differences in schizophrenic-type symptoms, but these are difficult to interpret. Suffice it to say that a larger number of depressive symptoms seem to make for a somewhat better prognosis as well as a negative family history of schizophrenia. These data, then, are similar to the data that have been reported by Stephens and co-workers (1960) and Vaillant (1964).

## The Concept of Sporadic Depressive Disease

Originally, in dealing with familial subtypes of depression, depression spectrum disease (depression with a family history of alcoholism) was separated from the remaining depressive. In most family history studies, however, the remainder may be divided into two groups: a larger group with no family history of any significant depressive illness and another group that has a history of depression only in the family. In the Iowa 500, there is evidence that the older the onset, the less likely there will be a positive family history of depression (Winokur 1979). Such negative family history depressive patients might be called "sporadic." In the Iowa 500, as in a series of other studies, sibships that are positive for depression are found more likely in those probands who have a family history of depression in other classes of relatives like parents. This suggests that older depressive patients with a negative family history may be showing a different illness from younger depressive patients. Of course, a perfectly legitimate alternative explanation is that the late onset depressive patients have a less severe illness and, consequently, are less likely to have a positive family history. This would be in favor of polygenic or multifactorial transmission of unipolar depression. However, it is not possible to separate this from the possibility that a sporadic depression is a separate and autonomous illness. There are certainly few data to support sporadic depression as an autonomous illness at this point, but it is worth another look. On the basis of a familial subtyping of depression, one could now divide pure depressive disease into familial pure depressive disease and sporadic depressive disease, the former having a family history of depression and the latter lacking this type of family background. Whether this would be a useful differentiation, however, awaits further research.

# Chapter 10

# The Gospel According to Fieldwork

## Methodology of Follow-Up and Epidemiologic Findings

By 1970, the appropriate way to study an illness was by a systematic evaluation. In all possible circumstances, the subjects were to be personally followed up and family studies were to include personal examinations of the relatives. In practice, this means that all people must be evaluated, and all people must be asked the same questions or subjected to exactly the same kind of tests. Interestingly, the pioneers in these kinds of systematic evaluations were the Scandinavians, who, because of manageable populations and disease registries, had accomplished very good follow-up studies. In general, their genetic and familial evaluations were accomplished by records, and the Iowa 500 made a serious effort to accomplish a true family study where the relatives were personally interviewed. The standard for a study of psychotic illness and the importance of genetic factors is the personal follow-up of cases and family members using a standardized instrument for gathering information. This is not to

181

imply that a study of records is not useful or informative, but the personal interview is absolutely necessary because often the records do not contain the answers to major questions and are not designed for research purposes. What they do have is as reliable as the personal interview, but they are by nature incomplete. Obtaining the personal interviews is scientifically sound and is accomplished by persistent and vigorous fieldwork.

## General Methodology

Simply stated, the objective of the fieldwork in the Iowa 500 was to interview all living patients, evaluate all records in both living and deceased patients, and systematically evaluate all first-degree family members who were available and willing to be interviewed. The interview that was used for these purposes was called the Iowa Structured Psychiatric Interview (ISPI) (Tsuang et al. 1980c). It was a standardized interview for trained nonmedical research workers that could be used to interview subjects blind to their clinical diagnosis or family status. Elaborate reliability and validity studies were performed using the ISPI.

Lifetime diagnoses of the interviewed subjects were made by staff psychiatrists based on completed ISPI interviews and on medical records if present. These medical records were relevant to subsequent admissions to any of the five state psychiatric hospitals in Iowa, which includes the Iowa Psychopathic Hospital—the site of the index admission. Two psychiatrists independently reviewed the interview forms, and the third psychiatrist compared the two diagnoses to make a consensus diagnosis. One psychiatrist used the Feighner criteria for a final diagnosis, and the other one used the criteria of the International Classification of Disease. If the first and second diagnoses were concordant, this became the final diagnosis. But if they were discordant, the diagnostic exercise was repeated by the first two psychiatrists. The third psychiatrist then made the final diagnosis by reviewing all information used by the first two raters. For classification and analysis purposes, the final diagnoses were coded numerically.

Patients who had died or who refused to be interviewed were given final diagnoses based on an "approximate" ISPI form by staff psychiatrists following the diagnostic procedures described above. These ISPI forms were completed by residents and physicians who reviewed all the medical records available on the deceased subjects and the subjects who refused to be interviewed and filled out the corresponding ISPI. This procedure was used both for first-degree family members as well as probands. Both the interviewers and the diagnosticians were blind to the research diagnoses of the index patients and the relationship of the subjects interviewed to the index patients. In fact, the diagnosticians did not even know if the given interview form was for an index patient or a relative.

A control group was also used in the study. This provided a baseline for comparison and was composed of patients who were free of psychiatric symptoms and who had been admitted to the same medical center during the same period of time for either an appendectomy or a herniorrhaphy. Of the 160 selected, 65 were male, and 95 were female. As discussed in Chapter 2, the selection of a control group made this a very unique study. Though we had a difficult time convincing the granting committee to fund us for a control group, it proved invaluable in the analysis stages. The control subjects allowed us to compare statistically our study groups to healthy subjects on the basis of family data, outcome, and mortality. The control subjects also added to the blindness aspect of the study. In all, we were able to trace 97% of the patients and control subjects to death or to current addresses (Tsuang et al. 1981b).

The ISPI is an interview form that was formulated for use in epidemiologic research in a general population as well as in a followed-up patient population (Tsuang et al. 1980c). The interview contains questions about the frequency and duration of symptoms that characterize schizophrenia, mania, depression, and neurosis. It can be used without any implication that either the informant or the informant's relatives have any type of psychiatric history or current psychiatric problems. As a starting point, the development of the ISPI used previously employed structured interview forms. The interview went through two drafts and was revised many times, resulting in a final version consisting of 235 questions covering the following areas: social history, alcohol and drug use, symptoms of schizophrenia, mania, depression and neurotic disorders, physical history, psychiatric treatment, and family history of psychiatric illness. The first effort at obtaining an estimate of reliability involved 20 screening questions where interviewers rated subjects one time each and different subjects were rated by different interviewers on two occasions. The screening questions for depression showed no disagreement. The results for the mania screening questions were less clear cut, although there was perfect agreement on the symptom "racing thoughts." The data suggested that symptoms of elation and pressure of speech were reliable but that the ratings for overactivity were not as reliable. All of the schizophrenia screening questions could be regarded as reliable and all of the neurosis screening questions were reliable except for those on compulsions. A similar reliability study was accomplished 4 years later showing that reliability was good for screening questions regarding depression, mania, and schizophrenia. Also, screening questions regarding neurosis were acceptably reliable but not as reliable as the questions for depression, mania, and schizophrenia. There was a series of behavioral items that was also investigated as to reliability. The total behavior ratings were found to be fairly reliable but not as reliable as the screening question ratings.

Validity was assessed on the 20 screening questions. There was a particular interest in the usefulness of the screening questions for eliciting reports of symptoms that differentiate people with severe psychiatric disorders from those who are labeled "psychiatrically normal." Also, the screening questions were used to identify for follow-up those people who shared common symptoms with diagnosed depressive, manic, schizophrenic, and neurotic patients. Both issues were investigated by using the fund of data amassed on 1,700 informants where interviews and hospital records were available. Without exception, the response rate for each screening question was higher for those with a positive psychiatric history. Also in the control group, a positive response rate was always less than 10% and, in fact, frequently zero. It was found that patients with depression had the highest response for depression screening questions. Patients with mania had the highest rate for mania screening questions, and schizophrenic patients had the highest rate for the schizophrenia screening questions in the follow-up interviews. The results for the neurosis screening questions were harder to interpret, although it was clear that control and manic subjects were less likely to respond to those items than depressive and schizophrenic patients and undiagnosed control subjects with a positive psychiatric history. Data on the groups of first-degree relatives of the manic, depressive, schizophrenic, and control subjects supported the expectations based on the assumed validity of the screening questions.

Validity was also measured by comparing the similarity between ratings by trained interviewers and criterion ratings made by qualified psychiatrists. On the whole, agreement on the screening questions was excellent, but agreement for the behavior ratings was weaker, although significantly greater than expected by chance in all cases. The conclusion that was drawn from the series of studies was that the screening questions for depression, mania, and schizophrenia could be utilized with confidence based on the results of the validity and interrater reliability. The reliability for the neurosis screening questions was lower than the reliability of the others, and the same pattern held for various studies of validity. Thus, the information about neurotic symptomatology would be less reliable than the information about the major psychoses. The individual behavior ratings were generally unreliable, mainly because these ratings must be based on subjective judgments of all behaviors exhibited during the interview, and, therefore, by themselves they are probably too unreliable for most research purposes.

The ISPI is divided into two parts. Part I deals with symptoms, age at which first noted, length of time the symptoms have been present, and how many periods of time in the individual's life that such symptoms might have occurred. These are the screening questions. Part I also contains a series of current manic and depressive symptoms asked of the patient and recorded by the interviewer; these questions are asked without any knowledge of the responses on Part II. Part II opens with schizophrenic symptoms currently experienced—simply their presence or absence. These are mainly symptoms of psychosis. Part II also includes a physical history, as well as the psychiatric history, which deals with number of hospitalizations and length and kinds of treatment on both an inpatient and outpatient basis. A family history is obtained in Part II. Finally, a behavior rating (current mental status) is completed after the interview.

## Some General Findings From the Field Study

One of the first and important sets of findings concerns the question of psychiatric disorders among the 160 surgical control patients (Tsuang et al. 1984). Table 10–1 shows the rates and morbidity risks of psychiatric disorders determined by the Feighner criteria in 541 relatives of controls where the proportions of ill relatives are given as a morbidity risk. The rates per 100 people, estimates that are often used, are generally lower as they are not controlled for age at risk. For rate estimates (rate per 100), people are counted as having fully gone through the age of risk. However, the findings are, in general, comparable. The morbid risk more closely approximates the actual risk for a psychiatric illness in a normal population. It should be noted that this population is a purified population (i.e., the control subjects are psychiatrically well and include no ill people, as far as it was able to be determined). An ordinary population would contain some psychiatrically ill patients, and, presumably, the relatives would then be slightly more likely to be ill. However, the differences will not be large in any event,

**Table 10–1.** Morbidity risks of psychiatric disorders in 541 relatives of control subjects

| Diagnosis | Males (N = 260) | | | Females (N = 281) | | | Total | | |
|---|---|---|---|---|---|---|---|---|---|
| | n | BZ | MR (%) | n | BZ | MR (%) | n | BZ | MR (%) |
| Schizophrenia | 0 | 227.5 | .0 | 0 | 245.0 | .0 | 0 | 472.4 | .0 |
| Mania | 0 | 159.0 | .0 | 3 | 185.0 | 1.6* | 3 | 344.0 | .9 |
| Depression | 6 | 159.0 | 3.8 | 22 | 185.0 | 11.9* | 28 | 344.0 | 8.1 |
| Neurosis | 5 | 227.5 | 2.2 | 7 | 245.0 | 2.9 | 12 | 472.5 | 2.5 |
| Personality disorder | 3 | 130.0 | 2.3 | 0 | 140.5 | .0* | 3 | 270.5 | 1.1 |
| Alcoholism | 15 | 223.5 | 6.7 | 1 | 239.5 | .4* | 16 | 463.0 | 3.5 |
| Drug abuse | 1 | 223.5 | .4 | 2 | 239.5 | .8 | 3 | 463.0 | .6 |
| Organic brain syndrome | 0 | 97.5 | .0 | 3 | 104.5 | 2.9 | 3 | 202.0 | 1.5 |
| Mental retardation | 0 | 130.0 | .0 | 0 | 140.5 | .0 | 0 | 270.5 | .0 |
| Undiagnosed and other disorders | 28 | 159.0 | 17.6 | 35 | 185.5 | 18.9 | 63 | 344.0 | 18.3 |
| No diagnosable mental disorder | 202 | — | — | 208 | — | — | 410 | — | — |

*Note.* BZ = number at risk; MR = morbidity risk that is the probability that a person will develop a specific disease at some time during his or her life, accounting for the manifestation period of the disease and the age of the person.
*P < .01 (comparison of females to males).

and we felt the relatives of the control subjects very closely approximated the general population.

In Table 10–1, the total (28 cases) for depression represents 18 definite, 7 probable, and 3 secondary cases. Mania includes two cases of definite depression with a history of mania and one case of definite mania. MR refers to the morbid risk and BZ refers to the number of people at risk, adjusted for age, at time of disappearance from observation. It is noteworthy that females are more likely to have a depression than males ($P =$ .01) and that males are more likely to have alcoholism than females ($P=$ .01). It is also notable that there are eight times as many depressive patients in the normal population than manic patients and that in this sample no control family member had schizophrenia. Interestingly, when one used less rigorous criteria (ICD-9), schizophrenia was seen in 0.6% of the population.

When ICD-9 criteria are used (World Health Organization 1978), the risks for depression and mania are slightly lower— 7.3% and 0.3%, respectively. In a recent epidemiologic study (L. Robins et al. 1984), the risks for depression (lifetime prevalence) range between 5.8% and 9.9% and, for mania, between 0.6% and 1.1%. This study and the Iowa 500 are not strictly comparable because of differences in criteria, racial composition, and urban-rural breakdown. Nevertheless, the differences are not all that great, suggesting that the purified control sample of the Iowa 500 probably reflected the general population, at least as far as mania and depression are concerned. Schizophrenia in the paper by L. Robins and co-workers was seen in 1.0%– 1.9% of the population, and this is higher than the 0.6% found in the Iowa 500 control subjects, even when the ICD-9 criteria were used.

As is often the case, the collection of large amounts of data lends itself to the solution of unforeseen questions. In particular, the study of the relatives of psychiatrically well control subjects allowed us to assess the occurrence of alcoholism in a sample of the nonpsychiatric population. Using the research criteria that were used in selecting the probands (Feighner et al.

1972), we found that it was possible to present morbidity risks for both men and women regarding alcoholism. The formula used to determine the number of people at risk was the Weinberg abridged method. MR was calculated according to the following formula, where $a$ is the number of affective individuals with alcoholism, $b$

$$MR = \frac{a}{b - b_o - \frac{1}{2}b_m}$$

the number of individuals examined, $b_o$ the number of individuals who have not yet reached the manifestation (risk) period, and $b_m$ the number of people who were in the middle of the risk period. The risk period for alcoholism was 20–39 years of age. An individual was considered to have alcoholism if he or she met the criteria at any time during his or her life, though he or she might be remitted at the time of the interview. Today, more sophisticated techniques such as life-table methodology would be used to calculate morbidity risks.

Table 10–2 presents the data (Winokur and Tsuang 1978). There were so few fathers and mothers who were interviewed that these data are not presented in the table. Most of the parents were deceased, a finding that is expected in that the control subjects were admitted to the hospital for surgical conditions from 1938–1948 and their relatives were examined in the 1970s. However, of three living fathers, none had alcoholism, and of 22 living mothers, none had alcoholism. The data in the table deal with siblings and children.

As one goes from definite criteria to definite and probable, there is an increase in the number of subjects with alcoholism. In this relatively modern sample, which was evaluated in the 1970s, the male alcoholic patients outnumber the female alcoholic patients by a factor of more than 10 to 1. These data are consistent with the study of Hagnell and Tunving (1972), who investigated the population of Lund in Sweden. The prevalence of alcoholism for men in that study was 10.3% and for women less than 1%. It is entirely possible that women may have the

**Table 10–2.** Rate and morbidity risk of alcoholism in 541 first-degree relatives of surgical control subjects using Feighner et al. diagnostic criteria

| | N | BZ | Definite Rate | Definite (%) | Definite and probable MR (%) | Rate | (%) | MR (%) |
|---|---|---|---|---|---|---|---|---|
| Men | 260 | 223.5 | 12 | (4.6) | 5.4 | 15 | (5.8) | 6.7 |
| Brothers | 123 | 121 | 6 | (5) | 5.0 | 8 | (6.5) | 6.6 |
| Sons | 134 | 99.5 | 6 | (4.5) | 6.0 | 7 | (5.2) | 7 |
| Women | 281 | 239.5 | 0 | (0) | .0 | 1 | (.4) | .4 |
| Sisters | 123 | 118.5 | 0 | (0) | .0 | 0 | (0) | .0 |
| Daughters | 136 | 99 | 0 | (0) | .0 | 1 | (.7) | 1 |

*Note.* BZ = number at risk; MR = morbidity risk.

same biological or familial propensity for alcoholism as men, but they may express this as a character disorder or a depressive neurosis or even possibly as a depressive psychosis. In comparison with the epidemiologic study of L. Robins and associates (1984), alcoholism seems underrepresented in the Iowa 500 control subjects, which may be due to population differences and differences in which symptoms constitute the criteria for the diagnosis of alcoholism.

Over the years, there have been reports of an association between schizophrenia and various medical illnesses and also between affective disorder and various physical diseases. Since our data represented long-term follow-up, a study of mortality was natural. Tsuang and co-workers (1983b) suggested that our data were such to warrant further studies of an increased incidence of gastrointestinal cancer, cardiovascular conditions, and infectious diseases in schizophrenia. Likewise, they suggested further studies on the possibilities of decreased incidence of lung cancer and rheumatoid arthritis in schizophrenia. In the major affective disorders, they suggested studies of increased incidence of circulatory, respiratory, and atopic diseases. Also, the data warranted further study of diabetes mellitus as particularly associated with affective disorder. Prior studies had methodological flaws, and the Iowa 500 with its long follow-up and meticulous accumulation of records lent itself to an evaluation of mortality. This project was one of the first in psychiatry to use newly developed statistical methodology.

Tsuang and Woolson (1977) evaluated the mortality data on schizophrenic, manic, and depressive patients, as well as 160 surgical control subjects (80 had appendectomies and 80 had herniorrhaphies). Data were available on 648 (95%) members of the study population. An age-sex standardized mortality ratio (SMR) was employed in order to express the mortality figures of the study population as compared with those of the state of Iowa, which, of course, was the geographic area from which the study group arose. Results were related to four decades, the first beginning in 1935 and ending in 1944, and the last ending in 1974. In no case did the control subjects ($n = 149$) have a significantly increased SMR (death rate). For the 99 schizophrenic males, there was an increased SMR in the first and second decade, but by the third and fourth decade this was not significantly increased. For the 93 schizophrenic females, there was a significant increase in death rate in the first, third and fourth decade of the study. For the manic patients ($n = 91$), no decade in the males was marked by a significant increase, but for the females there was a significant increase in SMR in the first and fourth decade. As regards the depressive patients ($n = 216$), both males and females had a significantly increased death rate in the first decade but no significant increase in the second, third, or fourth. The increased death rate was most pronounced in the first decade following admission although there were some exceptions (e.g., the schizophrenic females showed a significant increase even in the third and fourth decades).

## Natural (Medical) Causes of Death

In general, we know that psychiatric illnesses are clearly associated with unnatural deaths such as suicides and accidents. Nevertheless, a significant question exists as to whether or not psychiatric conditions bear some relationship to death from ordinary medical diseases. In other words, does an individual with schizophrenia, mania, or depression have an increased tendency to die from one or more specific medical diseases? A simple epidemiologic finding of an increase in death rate from natural causes would suggest further study into the why of the phenomenon and lend to a useful understanding of the nature of the psychiatric illnesses. Tsuang and Woolson (1978) excluded suicide and accidental deaths from the mortality analysis in order to determine whether death from natural causes in itself accounted for some of the excess mortality. They concluded that death, particularly in schizophrenia, due to suicides and accidental deaths was not the sole cause for excess mortality.

Tsuang and co-workers (1980a, 1980d, 1980e) noted a clearly decreased probability of surviving in the male and female schizophrenic, female manic, and male and female depressive patients. Specifically, this was a decreased probability of surviving 30 years after admission. There was a decrease in life expectancy of 9–10 years in schizophrenic, 14 years in female manic, and 7 years in the depressive patients. The absolute mortality for deaths due to cancer in the sample was not significantly different from that in the Iowa general population. However, the proportional mortality (see discussion below) showed a deficiency in deaths due to neoplasm in both schizophrenia and affective disorders, which may simply be due to the fact that there was a higher death rate early on from unnatural causes. Proportional mortality is the proportion of deaths due to a specific cause assessed against the total number of deaths from all causes.

More specifically, Tsuang and associates looked at death by neoplasms, diseases of the circulatory system, infections, and other causes. Circulatory system diseases included acute myocardial infarction and generalized ischemic cerebrovascular disease. Neoplastic diseases included lung cancer and skin cancer; infections included parasitic diseases, tuberculosis, poliomyelitis, syphilis; and other causes of death included respiratory, digestive, nervous system, genitourinary, and muscular-skeletal diseases. In schizophrenia, death from infection was increased both for males and females, and, for females, death from other causes was significantly increased. In mania, females showed increased death rates from circulatory system diseases. Depressed patients, either male or female, showed no increase in any of the causes of natural mortality. The increase in mortality in schizophrenia due to infectious diseases is a particularly interesting finding. Certainly, it has been attributed to the effects of long-term hospitalization; however, Lewis (1923) evaluated 403 autopsies of white schizophrenic males in a large psychiatric hospital. He noted that of these schizophrenic males, 315 (78%) had tuberculosis, and of 44 autopsies of white females, 77% showed tuberculosis. Similar findings were reported for black patients. This may be high even for chronically hospitalized patients who are living in crowded conditions and suggests that there may be something in schizophrenia that is relevant to a proclivity for developing severe infections and dying of them. However, at this point the why of the increased death rates from natural causes in general is shrouded in mystery.

Tsuang and co-workers (1980e) specifically evaluated deaths from cancer. In absolute mortality estimations (i.e., in comparison with the general population), there was no increase or decrease of deaths from neoplasm in schizophrenia. In a proportionate mortality analysis, one would divide the number of neoplastic deaths by the total number of deaths. In this case, there is a significant decrease in number of deaths in schizophrenia that might be attributed to neoplasm. However, as noted before, this smaller than expected proportional mortality probably is due to the fact that there is a large number of total deaths in schizophrenia, a very large proportion of these being unnatural causes such as suicides and accidents. There is a third method, the Cox regression model, which was used to compare the risk of dying of neoplasm in schizophrenia with the risk in surgical control subjects (Cox 1972). In this evaluation, the relative risk for neoplastic death in schizophrenia was significantly lower in comparison with the control group, but, in an evaluation of the control subjects, it was noted that they had more cancer deaths than the Iowa cancer rates predicted, and this might explain the deficiency in the schizophrenic patients. In any event, cancer mortality in schizophrenia is an area that may deserve somewhat more investigation.

## Deaths by Unnatural Causes (Suicide and Accident)

A long-term follow-up is a particularly good way to assess suicide in manic depression and schizophrenia because little speculative projection is necessary about what will happen to the rates in the future. In the first evaluation of the 30- to 40-year follow-up data for 76 manic, 182 depressive, 170 schizophrenic patients, and 109 control subjects, it was noted that 10% of the schizophrenic, 8.5% of the manic, and 10.6% of the depressive patients who were deceased had died by suicide; but none of the control subjects had committed suicide. There was a suggestion in the data that suicide occurred at an earlier age in schizophrenia than in the other psychiatric illnesses (Winokur and Tsuang 1975a).

Tsuang and Woolson (1978) added more data to the evaluation of suicide as well as material on accidental deaths. Table 10–3 gives the findings as a proportion of the deaths due to suicide and accidents of those who were deceased. When compared with the general population, data on male schizophrenic, female manic, and male and female depressive patients all showed a significant increase in suicide over what would be expected. Regarding accidents, female schizophrenic and male manic patients had a significant increase in expectancy over the general population. In female schizophrenic and male manic patients, there was an increase in observed over expected amounts of suicide, but this did not reach significance. Interestingly, accidental deaths were significantly higher in female schizophrenic and male manic patients, these two groups being the ones that did not show the increase in suicide. Thus, there is an increase in unnatural deaths in all three of the patient groups but no increase in the control group. Among the accidental deaths for the three psychiatrically ill groups, eight were considered deaths due to exhaustion. Also, of three deaths that had been signed out as accidents on the death certificates, fieldwork suggested that the true cause was suicide.

In the patient groups that had been followed for 30–40 years, it is notable that all three of the clinical groups have an increase in suicide rate and that the proportional increase in suicide rates (estimated as the number of deaths by suicide in those patients who were deceased) was about equal for schizophrenia, mania, and depression. Certainly, in a study of suicides

**Table 10–3.** Deaths by suicide and accident in schizophrenic, manic, depressive, and control subjects

| Diagnosis | N deceased | Suicides N (% deceased) | Accidents N (% deceased) | All unnatural deaths N (% deceased) |
|---|---|---|---|---|
| Schizophrenia | 78 | 7 (9) | 6 (7.7) | 13 (16.7) |
| Mania | 54 | 5 (9.3) | 5 (9.3) | 10 (18.5) |
| Depression | 162 | 13 (8) | 12 (7.4) | 25 (15.4) |
| Control subjects | 54 | 1 (1.9) | 0 (0) | 1 (1.9) |

in a population, schizophrenia is less likely to be diagnosed than affective disorder or alcoholism, but this may simply be due to the fact that schizophrenia is a less frequent disease than the affective disorders or alcoholism in the population (E. Robins et al. 1959).

# Chapter 11

# What the Future Held

## 30- to 40-Year Course and Outcome in Patients According to Final Diagnosis

> "The fair breeze blew,
> the white foam flew,
> The furrow followed free;
> We were the first that ever burst
> Into that silent sea . . ."
>
> —Samuel Taylor Coleridge,
> "The Rime of the Ancient
> Mariner"

The Iowa 500 was the first study that assessed the course and outcome in schizophrenia and the affective disorders after 30–40 years and anchored the findings to a systematic assessment at index admission.

As noted earlier, an evaluation of the stability of psychiatric diagnosis was made on the basis of the short-term chart follow-up. A similar assessment was made on the basis of the follow-up over 30–40 years (Tsuang et al. 1981a, 1981b), following two procedures. In the first case, we were able to assess the personal interview and determine whether or not the final diagnosis made by personal interview and assigned according to research criteria matched the original diagnoses made by research criteria at the beginning of the project. In the second methodology, one evaluated the stability of the diagnosis on the basis of medical records. This is necessary because a few people were unwilling to be interviewed, and many people were deceased by the time of the final assessment. Table 11–1 presents the stability of psychiatric diagnosis.

Regardless of the specific method used, it is clear that schizophrenia is quite stable. Ninety-three to 96% of the patients continued to have the diagnosis of schizophrenia. In the case of bipolar illness, 56%–80% of the patients continued to have the same diagnosis and, in the case of unipolar illness, 63%–84% of the patients. The stability of the schizophrenia was significantly higher than that of bipolar disorder or unipolar disorder at the 5% level of confidence, but no significant difference was found between the bipolar and unipolar disorders. The sta-

**Table 11–1.** Stability of psychiatric diagnosis of index diagnoses at follow-up

|  | Index diagnoses | | | |
|  | Schizophrenia | Bipolar | Unipolar | Control |
|---|---|---|---|---|
| **Personal interview** | | | | |
| Follow-up diagnoses | $N = 93$ | $N = 25$ | $N = 35$ | $N = 68$ |
|   Schizophrenia | 86 (93) | 2 (8) | 2 (6) | 0 (0) |
|   Bipolar | 2 (2) | 14 (56) | 6 (17) | 2 (3) |
|   Unipolar | 2 (2) | 5 (20) | 22 (63) | 4(6) |
|   Other | 3 (3) | 3 (12) | 5 (14) | 12(18) |
|   No mental disorder | 0 (0) | 1 (4) | 0 (0) | 50 (74) |
| **Medical records** | | | | |
| Follow-up diagnoses | $N = 81$ | $N = 46$ | $N = 108$ | $N = 1$ |
|   Schizophrenia | 78 (96) | 6 (13) | 5 (5) | 1 (100) |
|   Bipolar | 2 (3) | 37 (80) | 12 (11) | 0 (0) |
|   Unipolar | 0 (0) | 2 (4) | 91 (84) | 0 (0) |
|   Organic psychosis | 1 (1) | 1 (2) | 0 (0) | 0 (0) |

*Note.*  Values are $n$ (%).

bility is better where the material is based on medical records. A few patients go from bipolar to unipolar (a change of questionable validity), but more go from unipolar to bipolar, which creates some of the differences between the stability of the schizophrenic and the affective disorder groups. On the basis of personal interview, after adding together the bipolar and unipolar patients, we found that for the combined affective disorder group the stability was 78.3%, which was significantly different from the 93% of the schizophrenic groups at the 5% level. However, for those rated by records, the stability of the affective disorders was 92% versus the 96% in the schizophrenia group, which is comparable.

Of the 68 psychiatrically symptom-free controls, 73.5% received a diagnosis of no mental disorder. However, although these patients were selected specifically because they were free of psychiatric disorder, 27% earned a diagnosis in the 30- to 40-year follow-up. Of these, the largest number had a diagnosis of neurosis (9%); 3% had a diagnosis of personality disorder. This suggests that no matter how hard one tries, it is difficult, if not impossible, to select a psychiatric illness-free control group on the basis of records. In fact, the amount of psychiatric illness in the control group in follow-up is not all that different from other epidemiologic studies. Simply selecting a group based on having no obvious symptoms of a psychiatric nature, no record of illness, and no history of having taken medicine for "nervousness" does not seem to eliminate psychiatric illness. Even selecting a non-ill group by personal examination may be unreliable to some extent because people who are considered well may develop an illness in the follow-up. Also, all interviews may produce a small number of false negatives. The selection of the control groups for epidemiologic studies is a very important issue to consider when designing a study. The important point, however, is that the patients originally chosen by clear and unequivocal criteria continued in the main to have the same diagnosis.

Of 54 paranoid schizophrenic patients, 41% ultimately evolved into nonparanoid (hebephrenic-catatonic) schizophrenia. However, of 120 nonparanoid schizophrenic patients, only 10% were considered paranoid at the end of the follow-up. This strongly suggests that the evolution of schizophrenia may go from paranoid to nonparanoid but not the other way.

Thus, the diagnostic stability of schizophrenia and the affective disorders is quite good; data in the long-term follow-up were similar to the short-term follow-up that was published earlier (Winokur 1974a). This possibly suggests that stability assessed over a period of 2–5 years ought to be sufficient for a reliably diagnosed group to study.

## The Change From Unipolar Depression to Bipolar Illness

Of the 225 unipolar depressive patients who were admitted to the study, 22 became bipolar during the follow-up period with half of these occurring in the first few years. When comparing the 22 unipolar patients who became bipolar to the 203 stable unipolar patients, some differences at admission are notable. These are seen in Table 11–2 (Winokur and Wesner 1987). Those patients who became bipolar were younger, showed more self-reproach and guilt, had a longer index hospitalization, and also they were more likely men. There were some trends that separated the groups but did not reach significance. Regarding symptoms at index admission, unipolar patients who became bipolar, compared with stable unipolar patients, were more likely to suffer from early morning awakening (32% versus 16%), retardation (82% versus 60%), and decrease in concentration (73% versus 55%). They were also more likely to have had three or more episodes prior to index (14% versus 5%).

There are, then, some significant differences between stable unipolar patients and unipolar patients who become bipolar. In general, the positive findings are that those people who become bipolar have a history of more episodes in the past and a more positive family history for affective disorder as well as the pres-

ence of endogenous symptoms such as guilt, retardation, early
morning awakening, and concentration difficulties. Nevertheless,
such findings do not invariably predict a switch to bipolarity.

## Long-Term Outcome of Schizophrenia and the Affective Disorders

Schizophrenia classically differs from the affective disorders in
that it has a chronic, often deteriorating, course, and the affective disorders have an episodic course with a higher degree of
recovery. Certainly, if one looks at the short-term follow-up in a
previous chapter, these statements are supported. The outcome after a long period of follow-up is less well known, and we
are interested in how these disorders differ in their long-term
effect on hospitalized psychiatric patients who suffer from
schizophrenia, bipolar disorder, and unipolar disorder. With
this in mind, the investigators of the Iowa 500 assessed many of

**Table 11–2.**  Characteristics of unipolar patients who become
bipolar and stable unipolar patients

|  | Unipolar bipolar N = 22 | Stable unipolar N = 203 | P |
|---|---|---|---|
| n (%), male | 16 (73) | 85 (42) | .006 |
| Age < 30, n (%) | 7 (31) | 27 (13) | .025 |
| Marked self-reproach, guilt, n (%) | 21 (96) | 134 (66) | .04 |
| Proportion with affectively ill sisters, n (%) | 0 (0) | 35 (17) | .05 |
| Length of index hospitalization, ≥2 months, n (%) | 10 (45) | 39 (19) | .005 |
| Two or more subsequent hospitalizations, n (%) | 9 (41) | 29 (14) | .005 |

the former findings from previous outcome studies to determine the best methods to be used. In our study, not only are the
patients with different diagnoses compared with each other,
but they are also compared with a psychiatrically symptom-free
surgical control group that serves as a baseline for comparison.

Early on, the three patient groups were compared with each
other on the basis of employment status, physical health, and
mental health. Employment status was, at its best, working at
capacity or gainfully self-employed and, at its worst, unable to
work or incapacitated. For physical health, the ratings were
healthy to chronic illness, and, for mental health, the best rating was no indication of mental illness to obvious indication of
mental illness. For depression, 26% of the patients were considered severely disabled, and 46% had no disability at all. For mania, 29% were considered severely disabled, and 36% had no
disability. For schizophrenia, 48% were considered severely disabled, and 19% had no disability (Tsuang and Winokur 1975).
This is a somewhat less precise way to evaluate psychiatric disability than was done later on, but the findings are essentially
the same with schizophrenia appearing to be the most severely
disabled group of psychiatric patients.

Tsuang and co-workers (1979) looked at the patients of the
Iowa 500 after performing a 30- to 40-year field follow-up.
Operational criteria were presented to assess outcome on four
variables—marital, residential, occupational, and psychiatric
status. These outcome variables were evaluated by raters who
had no knowledge of the original diagnoses. Table 11–3 gives
the definition of outcome ratings; as may be noted, ratings were
good, fair, or poor. The statistical comparisons of outcomes for
each diagnostic category are presented in Figure 11–1.

Each of the ratings was assigned a number: good = 3,
fair = 2, and poor = 1. A combined mean outcome was assessed
for each of the four groups and was 1.80 for schizophrenic, 2.38
for manic, 2.42 for depressive, and 2.79 for control subjects. For
the combined outcome, schizophrenia was significantly poorer
when compared with the three remaining groups. Both mania
and depression were significantly poorer than the control group

for the combined outcome variable, but mania and depression were not significantly different from each other.

A fifth outcome variable was also analyzed. This is mortality, which was discussed previously. In summary, the control group shows no significant difference from the general Iowa population. For the affective disorders, the excess mortality relative to the general population of the state of Iowa disappeared after the first decade of the follow-up, but, for schizophrenia, the excess mortality persisted over the 30-plus year follow-up period.

Of particular interest are the proportions of patients that were asymptomatic at follow-up. These patients were rated as having no psychiatric symptoms: for schizophrenia 38 of 186 (20%), for mania 43 of 86 (50%), and for depression 129 of 212 (61%). The control subjects as expected were overwhelmingly asymptomatic (122 of 144; 85%). There were 38 schizophrenic patients (20%) who were asymptomatic, but larger numbers of schizophrenic patients had a good outcome status on occupational (65; 35%) and residential (64; 34%) items. This suggests a possible dissociation between clinical symptomatology and psychosocial disability over time. Marital status paralleled clinical status with a rating of good seen in 21% of the cases.

**Table 11–3.** Outcome ratings of patients and control subjects

| Status | Good | Fair | Poor |
|---|---|---|---|
| Marital | Married or widowed | Divorced or separated | Single, never married |
| Residential | Own home or relative's residence | Nursing or county home | Mental hospital |
| Occupational | Employed, retired, home-maker, or student | Incapacitated due to physical illness | Incapacitated due to mental illness |
| Psychiatric symptoms | None | Some | Incapacitating |

*Source.* Adapted from Tsuang et al. 1979.

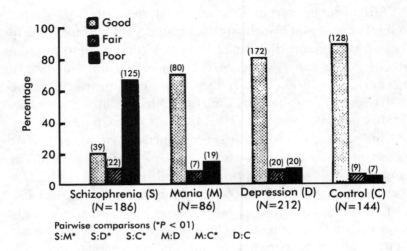

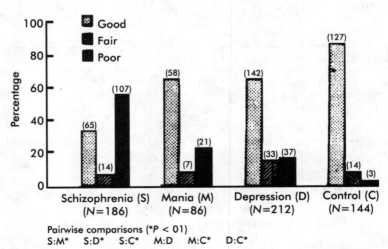

**Figure 11–1.** Percentage of outcome status variables by diagnostic *groups.*
*Source.* Adapted from Tsuang et al. 1979.

# Residential Status

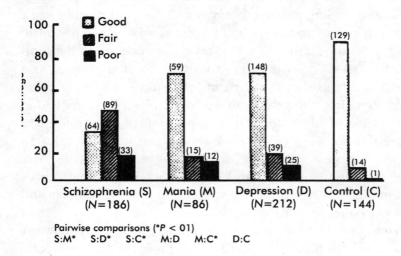

Pairwise comparisons (*P < 01)
S:M*    S:D*    S:C*    M:D    M:C*    D:C

# Psychiatric Status

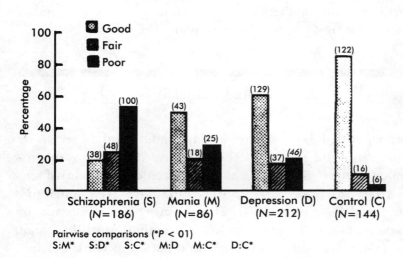

Pairwise comparisons (*P < 01)
S:M*    S:D*    S:C*    M:D    M:C*    D:C*

Tsuang and co-workers (1979) were aware that some of the selection criteria might influence the outcome, specifically in schizophrenia. Single marital status and poor premorbid work history both were parts of the criteria that might have influenced the follow-up findings. However, the authors used a multivariate analysis of covariance to adjust for the marital and occupational status at the time of follow-up. This was accomplished by using the covariants of marital and occupational status at time of admission. The comparisons of the outcome in these measures were made after this adjustment in order to avoid the inherent criteria biases for the outcome study. The outcome was unchanged from that presented in the four figures shown in Figure 11–1, the highest being in control subjects and the lowest being in schizophrenic subjects.

An additional factor was that the Feighner criteria demand at least 6 months of illness in order for a diagnosis of schizophrenia. However, 80% of the schizophrenia group were composed of first-admission patients, and this would obviate the effect of duration as assessed by previous hospitalization on the outcome. Further, the follow-up was 30–40 years, and it would appear that the 6-month criterion predicts a poor outcome after a considerable length of time, not just a short-term poor outcome.

## Long-Term Outcome and Schizoaffective Disorder

Earlier, we noted 315 patients who had a hospital diagnosis of schizophrenia did not meet the Feighner criteria for schizophrenia. Of these, 85 had both schizophrenic and affective features that provided a group of "schizoaffective" patients (Tsuang and Dempsey 1979). The mean age at admission of these patients was 29 years, which is exactly that of the mean age of admission of the schizophrenic patients. On the other hand, the manic patients were 34, the depressive patients were 44, and the control subjects were 32 years at admission. These 85 schizoaffective patients were traced, and for 99% of those traced (73 of 74), there was sufficient information to rate all four outcome variables. Based on the variable of marital status, the schizoaffective patients were significantly better than the schizophrenic patients and significantly worse than the control subjects but not significantly different from the manic and depressive patients. Based on the variable of residential status, the same findings pertained. Based on their occupational status, schizoaffective patients were not significantly different from the schizophrenic or manic patients but significantly less well off than the depressive and control subjects. Regarding psychiatric status, schizoaffective subjects were not significantly different from the those with schizophrenia but significantly worse than the manic, depressive, or control subjects. Finally, on the combined outcome, patients who were schizoaffective were better than the schizophrenic patients but worse than the manic, depressive, and control subjects. The findings suggest that schizoaffective disorder has a significantly better outcome than schizophrenia but a poorer outcome than the affective disorder and control subjects. The meaning of these findings is not readily evident. It is possible that schizoaffective disorder, as it was defined, includes a mixed group of patients, some suffering from schizophrenia and others from affective disorders. Another possibility exists, which is that there is another autonomous disorder with components of each and an outcome that falls between the two illnesses. Related to the first possibility is that the diagnosis of schizoaffective disorder may identify patients who are difficult to diagnose but who, nevertheless, constitute a mixed group of patients with schizophrenia and affective disorder of unknown proportions.

## Factors Leading to Good and Poor Outcome

Tsuang and colleagues (1981a) additionally used the outcome assessment in Table 11–3 to separate disorders based on admission information. Discounting marital status, they dichotomized the three remaining outcome variables using poor outcome versus others, good and fair. With this method, they confirmed previous findings (i.e., a poor outcome in schizophrenia was found in comparison with the affective disorders, and no differences were seen between mania and depression). They then looked at some of the index variables in order to determine whether any of these might be associated with a poor outcome. Within schizophrenia, disorganized thoughts at index admission was associated with a poor outcome, but a better outcome was associated with the presence of delusions or hallucinations. Within the affective disorders, bipolar patients with grandiose delusions or ideas showed a poor outcome. A better outcome was found in depressive patients of a unipolar type who had complaints of fatigue or tiredness at the time of index admission. These authors took the schizophrenia findings as evidence of support of the idea of a subdivision of schizophrenia into paranoid and nonparanoid types (Tsuang and Winokur 1974). The delusions and hallucinations were ordinarily associated with paranoid schizophrenia and hebephrenic-catatonic schizophrenia, and it was only with the addition of disorganized thoughts that the person was able to be called nonparanoid. Thus, on the basis of the long-term outcome, the findings do support a difference between paranoid and nonparanoid schizophrenia. However, there were no differences of any note between the paranoid and nonparanoid schizophrenic patients on the variable of familial schizophrenia, which was assessed by the blind family studies; this would be against confirmation of this kind of subdivision in schizophrenia (Tsuang et al. 1980b).

## The Evolution of Symptoms in Hebephrenic-Catatonic Schizophrenia

Hebephrenic and catatonic symptoms go together in the same person (Böök 1953; Tsuang and Winokur 1974), and, with a long-term follow-up and good access to records, it is possible to evaluate the evolution of these specific symptoms. Pfohl and Winokur (1982a, 1982b, 1983) accomplished this by separating the charts of 52 hebephrenic-catatonic schizophrenic patients requiring long-term hospitalization from the group of Iowa 500 patients. Presence or absence of 28 different symptoms was noted on a year-by-year basis over a period of 35 years. The age at onset of these patients was 21 years, and they had been ill for an average of 2.5 years from onset to index hospitalization. The duration of the follow-up was 30 years, and these patients were 54 years old at the time of last follow-up. They had an average of 2.8 hospitalizations, and the mean number of hospitalizations until chronic institutionalization was 1.6. The mean number of episodes was 1.7; 20 of the 52 patients had at least a partial remission after the initial onset of symptoms during which time they were able to return to some form of independent living; 6 of the 20 were described by family and professionals as having a remission during which they were completely back to normal. The remissions almost always occurred within a year after the onset. However, all 52 of the patients (100%) were eventually chronically institutionalized, and none had the benefit of psychotropic medication at any point in the short-term follow-up. During or before the year of first hospitalization, certain symptoms were noted to be quite likely present. Productivity of less than 50%, lack of volition, inappropriate affect, loose association of thoughts, persecutory delusions, other delusions, and auditory hallucinations were common and were individually present in 75%–100% of the patients at some time during the illness; however, it should be noted that these symptoms were present earlier. There was a second group of symptoms that had their onset at around 5 or more years after the first hospitalization. These included impaired self-care, severely impaired social interaction, inability to do any work, hypoactivity, waxy flexibility, mannerisms, flat affect, decreased speech, incoherent speech, and sensorium defects. In over 50% of the patients who had originally had them, the symptoms that tended to disappear included severely impaired self-care, waxy flexibility, bizarre behavior, tics and grimaces, elevated mood, depressed mood, persecutory delusions, grandiose delusions, auditory hallucinations, and first-rank symptoms. It should be noted that these symptoms had disappeared before the advent of phenothiazines. Interestingly, 16 of the 52 patients had depressed mood, which occurred early in the course, and all but 1 subsequently lost it. Inappropriate affect was found in 42 of the 52 patients, and 19 of these eventually lost the inappropriate affect, which was usually replaced by flatness of affect. All of the patients had flat affect or inappropriate affect at some time during the course of their illness, but this was a symptom generally required for the diagnosis of hebephrenic-catatonic schizophrenia (Tsuang and Winokur 1974). Symptoms generally classified as positive symptoms of schizophrenia, such as hallucinations and delusions, were found to have an early onset, a tendency to resolve over time, a greater tendency to resolve than symptoms usually classified as negative symptoms (such as flat affect), decreased social interaction, and sensorium defects. In particular, avolition became increasingly frequent with the passage of time.

Most of the schizophrenic patients in this study of hebephrenic-catatonic schizophrenia had very poor insight in their first year of illness, and the level of insight decreased further over the next 5 years. Although many had an unremarkable premorbid personality, a substantial number of these patients did have a diagnosable personality disorder (18 of 52), and, of these 18, 8 could be diagnosed as having a schizoid personality disorder. Some authors have suggested that many of the symptoms of chronic schizophrenia might be ameliorated by manipulations in the institutional environment, but several lines of evidence suggest that the observations were not an artifact of institutionalization. Most of the symptoms reported began in a number of patients before the first hospitalization and simply intensified with time. Further, similar disabling symptoms have been reported in schizophrenic patients who have been engaged in very active programs of educational and social enrichment and also in schizophrenic patients who live in the community (Cheadle et al. 1978; Morgan 1979).

One hundred-thirty nonparanoid patients (mainly hebe-phrenic-catatonic) were compared with a group of 62 patients who had a diagnosis of paranoid schizophrenia at time of admission. At follow-up, 29 still had a diagnosis of paranoid schizophrenia (Winokur et al. 1987). There were some differences, such as the paranoid patients were older (34 versus 26 years) at admission and the paranoid patients were hospitalized 40 days at index admission as compared with the nonparanoid patients being hospitalized 50 days. Cause of death differences were that 11 of the 49 deceased nonparanoid patients died as a result of infectious diseases as opposed to 0 of 29 of the deceased paranoid patients. More of the paranoid patients were deceased at follow-up (49% versus 36%), but then this would be expected as they were older at time of admission. The most interesting point is the difference in cause of death, with infectious diseases looming large in the nonparanoid group. These data are not controlled for amount of hospitalization at follow-up; they do, however, suggest the possibility that patients with hebephrenic-catatonic schizophrenia in the past may have handled infection in a different way than other kinds of schizophrenic patients. Chronic institutionalization, poor nutrition, or less medical care could have contributed to the increased number of fatal infections. It is clear that hebephrenic-catatonic schizophrenic patients as they age become less of a problem in terms of active or positive symptomatology and more of a problem in terms of passive or negative symptoms. Thus, they may require a different kind of management than was necessary when they were younger.

## Subtyping Schizophrenias According to Outcome

Considerable research in psychiatry leads one to suspect that typical schizophrenia may be heterogeneous, which is supported by the increased frequency of schizophrenic syndromes associated with several medical and neurologic diseases (Davison 1983). Starting with Kraepelin, psychiatry worked with a tripartite division of schizophrenia into paranoid, hebephrenic, and catatonic, and, later, Bleuler added simple schizophrenia to the subtypes. In the stability study of psychiatric diagnosis, Tsuang and colleagues (1981b) noted that 41% of the paranoid schizophrenic patients changed subtype diagnoses, but only 10% of the nonparanoid hebephrenic-catatonic schizophrenic patients changed to the subtype diagnosis of paranoid schizophrenia. We should note, however, that 60% of the paranoid schizophrenic patients not only did not change subtype diagnosis, but, in general, they had a better course and outcome.

Tsuang (1982) noted that one variable identified poor outcome in three categories: marital status, occupational status, and presence of psychiatric symptoms. This one variable was the presence of memory deficit at index admission, which was defined as signs of disorientation and symptoms of recent or remote memory impairment. As the criteria for selection of the schizophrenic probands in the Iowa 500 excluded acute schizophrenia, the acute confusional state that is sometimes associated with acute psychosis was absent. In addition, these memory deficits were present without clouding of consciousness. These findings are important because, of the 22 patients who originally presented signs of memory deficit, 20 received a chart diagnosis of nonparanoid schizophrenia. At follow-up, 20 remained nonparanoid, which suggests that schizophrenic patients with memory deficit are still nonparanoid even 30–40 years after admission.

The memory deficit remained stable as shown by the fact that at follow-up, 30–40 years later, 43% of the patients with memory deficit at admission (assessed by mental status examination) still complained of impaired memory, but only 22% of the patients in the group without memory deficit complained of impaired memory. At follow-up, there was no difference in mean age for both groups, the average being 53 years. In the memory deficit group, 62% were disoriented compared with only 23% of the group that did not have memory deficit at admission. A comparison of rates of mortality at follow-up in patients with and without memory deficit revealed that the numbers of survival years were similar, which suggested that the memory deficit at admission of schizophrenic patients had a prognosis that differed from that seen in the common organic brain syndromes where the number of survival years is decreased.

Kendler and co-workers (1984) made a broad attempt to assess the outcome of schizophrenic subtypes defined by four separate diagnostic systems. Specifically, these systems were the DSM-III, the Research Diagnostic Criteria (RDC [Spitzer et al. 1978]), and the ICD-9 criteria (World Health Organization 1978) to which they added the Tsuang and Winokur criteria (1974), which separates hebephrenic-catatonic (nonparanoid) from paranoid schizophrenia. Two types of outcome were assessed: a short-term outcome coded as recovered/improved versus unrecovered based on chart information, with the mean length of follow-up being 2.5 years. Long-term outcome was determined by the follow-up in the field where the median length of long-term follow-up was 30 years, and the mean length was 24.1 years. Specifically, three dimensions of long-term outcome were evaluated: residential, occupational, and psychiatric, which were dichotomized into worse and better. For residential status, worse meant that the individual was residing in a nursing home, county home, or mental hospital, and better indicated that the followed-up patient was residing in his or her own or a relative's home. Occupational status was assessed as worse if the individual was incapacitated by mental illness but better if the person was employed, retired but active, a homemaker, or incapacitated by physical illness. Finally, psychiatric status was worse if the individual had incapacitating symptoms but better if there were no symptoms or only some nonincapacitating symptoms.

All of the diagnostic systems successfully separated the outcome in the paranoid and nonparanoid groups. The most successful system, however, turned out to be the Tsuang and Winokur criteria. For the short-term outcome, the Tsuang and Winokur criteria clearly showed a significantly better outcome for the paranoid rather than the hebephrenic-schizophrenic patients. The undifferentiated group in the Tsuang and Winokur criteria was not significantly different, however, from either the hebephrenic or the paranoid groups. Table 11–4 presents the material on long-term follow-up and the use of the Tsuang and Winokur criteria. Notably, residential and occupational status was better at differentiating the groups than psychiatric symptomatology. The differences between the hebephrenic and undifferentiated groups for the three variables were not significant, but the differences between the paranoid and hebephrenic groups always showed a significant difference. The patients in this sample, of course, were all selected by definition for the presence of symptoms that had lasted at least 6 months.

The difference, therefore, in outcome between paranoid and nonparanoid schizophrenic patients could not have resulted from inclusion of prognostically favorable acute schizophrenia, which often manifests itself by paranoid symptoms. However, there is one caveat that must be remembered; that is, the criteria used did not differentiate the patients with delusional disorder from those with schizophrenia. Some members of the paranoid group may well have had delusional disorder, which in general probably causes less deterioration occupationally and residentially (Opjordsmoen 1989). However, this admixture of delusional disorder (paranoia patients) with paranoid schizophrenia is unlikely to have accounted for the very marked differ-

**Table 11–4.**  Long-term outcome in paranoid versus hebephrenic versus undifferentiated schizophrenic patients: the Tsuang and Winokur criteria

| Residential outcome | Occupational outcome | Psychiatric outcome |
|---|---|---|
| P vs. H, $P = .001$ | P vs. H, $P = .01$ | P vs. H, $P = .05$ |
| P vs. U, $P = .01$ | P vs. U, $P = .05$ | P vs. U, $P = $ NS |
| H vs. U, $P = $ NS | H vs. U, $P = $ NS | H vs. U, $P = $ NS |

*Note.*   P = paranoid ($N = 33$); H = hebephrenic ($N = 40$); U = undifferentiated ($N = 102$); NS = not significant.

ences in outcome between the paranoid and nonparanoid groups, as the delusional disorder diagnosis accounted for very few patients. Kendler and co-workers (1984) note that the difference in outcome between paranoid and nonparanoid schizophrenia in all diagnostic systems was more noticeable at long-term than short-term outcome. This is possibly the result of deterioration in the nonparanoid group as opposed to relative stability in the paranoid group. The findings clearly suggest that subtyping patients on the basis of systematic criteria applied to admission, and on the basis of the chart material, is predictive of the outcome measures, and, therefore, these data show considerable validity for the criteria. This outcome evaluation has the benefits of specific criteria-based diagnoses, a long follow-up period, and clearly defined outcome measures, all of which may account for the success in separating the groups.

# Chapter 12

## Familial Psychiatric Illness in Schizophrenia and the Affective Disorders

### Psychiatric Illness in Relatives

> "This Nymph, that gazed upon his clustering locks,
> With ivy berries wreathed, and his blithe youth,
> Had by him, ere he parted thence, a son
> Much like his father but his mother more, . . ."
>
> —John Milton, "Comus"

One of the two main goals of the Iowa 500 study was to systematically evaluate the presence of psychiatric illness in family members of probands with depression, mania, and schizophrenia. We used systematic criteria of Feighner and colleagues (1972), and we planned to use the same criteria for the assessment of the relatives. In the case of schizophrenia, there was a problem since Feighner criteria included a family history of schizophrenia as one of the options in favor of the diagnosis in the proband. We removed this criterion because it was obvious to us that if we used it there would be a confounding factor. If schizophrenia were highly represented in family members (Tsuang et al. 1978), using a positive family history as a criterion for schizophrenia would predict a high rate of schizophrenia in the family. The family history of schizophrenia criterion was then replaced by the term "blunted affect," which was not in the original Feighner criteria. After a year of development and standardization, we had the instrument that was used for the family study, which was the Iowa Structured Psychiatric Interview (ISPI) (Tsuang et al. 1980c) described earlier. We were fortunate to have access to extremely detailed family records from the hospital charts and were able to do a good job of identifying and finding family members.

Prior research on bipolar illness (Winokur et al. 1969) had suggested that inquiring about a family history would yield very few false positives but many false negatives (around 22%). In other words, few ill relatives by family history were found to be well by personal examination, but many relatives thought to be well by family history were found to have had an illness when they were personally examined. This finding suggested that the appropriate way to study family background, and assess the possible genetic contribution, was to do a family study rather than simply a family history study. A family study, of course, is defined as a methodology in which all available first-degree family members are systematically interviewed in order to make a diagnosis.

We were able to trace 97% of the probands, and we were able to trace 90% of a total of 4,094 relatives. This was done through medical records, telephone, and personal interviews (Tsuang et al. 1980b). Of those traced, 55% were still alive, and it was possible to personally interview 1,578 (77%) of those using the structured interview, with the mean ages of those interviewed ranging from 49.8–60.6 years. As most schizophrenic patients never married, their first-degree relatives were mainly (and usually) siblings and parents. The mean age of their relatives, therefore, was greater than those of the relatives of the affective disorder groups and surgical control patients for whom mostly siblings and children were interviewed. A very positive aspect of the study was that most of the relatives had passed through the risk periods for schizophrenia and the affective disorders.

The interviewers were trained and sent into the field to interview living relatives. We also searched for records belonging to relatives who were deceased. If a hospital record of a deceased relative was available, a psychiatric resident was asked to complete the same structured interview form using information from the hospital record, which we called the "approximate ISPI." ISPI was used for the personal assessments. In total, there were 70 approximate ISPIs for the deceased relatives.

The diagnoses were arrived at by having two psychiatrists review the assessment interview; one used the Feighner criteria, and the other used ICD-9 as a basis for making a diagnosis. If two independent diagnoses were concordant, this became the final diagnosis, but if the independent diagnoses were discordant after this process was completed, and if it still turned out to be discordant after discussion, a third psychiatrist made the final diagnosis by a systematic review of all available material.

Tables 12–1 and 12–2 present the material from the personal interviews of the first-degree relatives of the four original diagnostic groups. The diagnoses of the family members were the final diagnoses after all of the diagnostic negotiating had occurred. The evaluation of schizophrenia in first-degree relatives is presented in Table 12–1. As expected, the family history

**Table 12–1.** Morbidity risks of schizophrenia in personally interviewed primary relatives of patients with schizophrenia, mania, depression, and surgical conditions (control subjects)

| | Number interviewed | Schizophrenia (%) | At risk | Morbid risk (% ± SE) |
|---|---|---|---|---|
| Schizophrenia (S) | 354 | 11 (3.1) | 346 | 3.2 ± .94 |
| Mania (M) | 216 | 2 (.9) | 204 | 1 ± .69 |
| Depression (D) | 467 | 4 (.9) | 435 | .9 ± .46 |
| Control (C) | 541 | 3 (.6) | 473 | .6 ± .37 |

*Note.* Pairwise comparisons: S:M[*]; S:D[**]; S:C[**]; M:D; M:C; D:C.
[*]$P < .10$; [**]$P < .05$.
*Source.* Adapted from Tsuang et al. 1980b.

for schizophrenia was higher in the relatives of schizophrenic probands than in the relatives of depressed, manic, or control probands. Schizophrenia in the relatives of manic, depressive, and control subjects did not differ from each other. Table 12–2 shows similar comparisons for affective disorder in the relatives. Affective disorder was significantly higher in the relatives of manic and depressive patients when compared with the relatives of schizophrenic or control subjects. Schizophrenic and control subjects did not differ from each other for the morbidity risk of affective disorder. The diagnoses for the relatives were made blind to the diagnosis of the probands. Also, the interviewers who went into the field to interview relatives did not have knowledge of the diagnosis of the proband. Interestingly, if one compares the data from the personal interviews with the family history material presented in an earlier chapter, one may note that they are not that much different. Surprising is the fact that the difference between affective disorder in relatives of schizophrenic patients versus relatives of affective disorder probands may be slightly higher in the family history study when compared with the family study data, which depended on the personal interviews.

**Table 12–2.** Affective disorder (mania and/or depression) in personally interviewed primary relatives of patients with schizophrenia, mania, depression, and surgical control subjects

|  | Number interviewed | Affective disorder (%) | At risk | Morbid risk (% ± SE) |
|---|---|---|---|---|
| Schizophrenia (S) | 354 | 19 (5.4) | 273 | 7 ± 1.54 |
| Mania (M) | 216 | 21 (9.7) | 160 | 13.1 ± 2.67 |
| Depression (D) | 467 | 44 (9.4) | 341 | 12.9 ± 1.82 |
| Control (C) | 541 | 26 (4.8) | 344 | 7.6 ± 1.43 |

*Note.* Pairwise comparisons: S:M[*]; S:D[**]; S:C; M:D; M:C[*]; D:C.[**]
[*]$P < .10$; [**]$P < .05$.
*Source.* Adapted from Tsuang et al. 1980b.

In the record evaluation for familial schizophrenia, the data are striking, showing that of 21 records of family members of schizophrenia patients, 9 diagnoses (42.9%) of schizophrenia were made. Of 47 records of the affective disorder patients, only 19% were blindly given the diagnosis of schizophrenia. Of two records that were available of family members of the control subjects, none were given a schizophrenia diagnosis. For family members of the nonschizophrenic probands, the highest proportion of records that were diagnosed as indicating schizophrenia in a relative was found in the mania group, 5 of 14 (36%).

## Familial Psychiatric Illness in Relatives of Manic and Depressed Patients

The previous section refers to the family study material for which researchers used the original diagnoses as a basis for separating the groups into schizophrenic, manic, and depressive. This poses a methodological problem in the case of the affective disorders in that 22 patients changed diagnosis, going from unipolar to bipolar at follow-up. This increased the size of the bipolar group by 22% and decreased the size of the unipolar group by 10%, which meant an appropriate assessment of psychopathology was needed to take these changes into account.

A first evaluation of familial affective disorder (based on personal interview and record searches) in 122 bipolar, 203 unipolar, and 160 control subjects revealed that among 666 relatives of bipolar patients there were 40 affective disorder (6%) diagnoses. Of 1,137 relatives of unipolar patients, 56 had a diagnosis of affective disorder (4.9%), and of 1,000 relatives of controls, 27 had an affective disorder diagnosis (2.7%). The control relatives differ from the bipolar relatives on the morbidity risk of affective disorder beyond the .001 level of probability, and they differ from the relatives of unipolar patients at the .01 level of probability. A diagnostic assessment was also made on the mental hospital records of relatives found in the three groups. For

122 bipolar probands, 17 records on relatives were found or .14 per proband; for 203 unipolar probands, 30 records were found or .15 per proband, and for 160 control probands, only two records were found or .01 records per proband (Winokur et al. 1981). Though the diagnoses of affective disorder determined by interview were twice as high in the relatives of bipolar and unipolar than control subjects, the existence of mental hospital records is 14–15 times higher in relatives of bipolar and unipolar disorder patients than in relatives of control subjects. Table 12–3 presents the morbid risks for affective disorder in the relatives of the three proband groups. The morbid risks for relatives of bipolar probands and unipolar probands are both significantly higher than the morbid risks in relatives of control probands (Winokur et al. 1982). Almost all of the diagnoses of unipolar depression in the relatives were based on personal interview, which was true of 89% of the affectively ill relatives of bipolar probands, 92% of the affectively ill relatives of unipolar probands, and 96% of the affectively ill relatives of the control probands. On the other hand, personal interviews appeared to miss bipolarity in relatives (Tsuang et al. 1981b) as is shown in Table 12–4, which shows morbidity risks based on chart material. It is noteworthy that bipolar probands were more likely than unipolar or control probands to have had bipolar relatives. As expected also, affective illness in relatives of unipolar was more

**Table 12–3.** Morbidity risks for affective disorder in personally examined primary relatives of bipolar (manic), unipolar depressed, and control subjects

| Proband group | Family members interviewed N | Ill with affective disorder N (%) | Family members at risk N (%)[a] | Morbid risk % ± SE |
|---|---|---|---|---|
| Bipolar (N = 122) | 267 | 28 (11) | 196 | 14.3 ± 2.50 |
| Unipolar (N = 203) | 416 | 37 (9) | 305 | 12.2 ± 1.87 |
| Control (N = 160) | 541 | 26 (5) | 344 | 7.6 ± 1.43 |

[a]Age of risk, 15–59 years.

frequently unipolar than bipolar. Again, one notes that the charts themselves seem to have more resolving power in separating groups than do the personal interviews. For the family study (personal examination) assessment, the ratio of ill first-degree relatives in the probands with bipolar or unipolar illness to the relatives of controls is less than two (13%–7.6%). Not only are there more charts per subject available for the bipolar and unipolar proband relatives, but the specific diagnoses are higher. For the bipolar and unipolar probands, there are 31 charts of deceased relatives that carry the diagnosis of mania and/or depression; for the control probands, there is one such chart. The ratio on the basis of charts per subject between the affectively ill probands and control probands is 9.5%–.3% or 31. Thus, there is approximately 1 of 10 probands who has a relative with a chart diagnosis of affective disorder in the bipolar patients and approximately 1 of 10 of the unipolar probands who has a relative with a chart diagnosis. On the other hand, only 1 of 160 control probands has an affective disorder relative by chart diagnosis. These findings suggest that a family history of a serious illness, which necessitates hospitalization, is a far better discriminator in separating affectively ill probands from control probands than a diagnosis made by personal interview (Winokur 1983).

If a person has a mental health record, he or she is, by definition, probably ill and will receive a psychiatric diagnosis. In the case of the relative of an affective disorder proband, that

**Table 12–4.** Bipolar or unipolar diagnosis from records of deceased primary relatives in three proband groups

| Proband group | Total deceased | Available charts $n$ (%) | With bipolar illness $n$ (%) | With unipolar illness $n$ (%) |
|---|---|---|---|---|
| Bipolar ($N = 122$) | 312 | 17 (5.4) | 8 (47) | 4 (24) |
| Unipolar ($N = 203$) | 606 | 30 (5) | 6 (20) | 13 (43) |
| Control ($N = 160$) | 322 | 2 (0.6) | 0 (0) | 1 (50) |

diagnosis will most likely be that of mania or depression. However, there is no *a priori* reason for the illness in the family member to lead to a hospitalization except for two possibilities: 1) having had a proband hospitalized may sensitize the family to seek hospitalization because of a previously successful outcome, and 2) what is transmitted in the family is severity as well as the presence of a specific illness. The differing levels of confidence in separating affective disorder probands from the control probands on the basis of a family history between the personal interview methodology, which includes only the presence of a syndrome, and the methodology that includes hospitalization as well as the presence of a syndrome suggest the need for some estimate of severity in diagnostic criteria.

Looking only at depression, we found that there were more women than men among the unipolar depressed relatives but equal numbers of men and women who were affectively ill among the bipolar relatives. Among relatives in all proband groups, including the schizophrenic group, depression was more frequent in females (59% for the schizophrenic group, 69% for the bipolar group, and 72% for the unipolar group). For control subjects, however, the finding was even more striking. Of 26 depressed relatives of the control subjects, 24 (92%) were women. These results indicate that it may be possible that there is a depressive illness in women that may not necessarily be related genetically or familially to bipolar illness or to unipolar illness. Thus, a preponderance of depressed women in a family study, particularly a family study of bipolar illness, might constitute a contamination, making it difficult to assess true familial transmission.

These findings suggest a sex polarity effect (Winokur and Crowe 1983). There were 40 affectively ill relatives of bipolar probands in the Iowa 500 study. Of these, 15% were bipolar males, 13% were bipolar females, 22% were unipolar males, but 50% were unipolar females. In assessing 14 studies of bipolar index patients, more unipolar depression than mania was found in women in 13 of the 14 studies, and more unipolar depression was found in female than in male relatives in 13 of the 14 studies. Two studies of control populations, one of which is the Iowa 500 and the other which is a segment of a collaborative study of affective disorder, show a marked excess (70%–92%) of depressive subjects being female. This too suggests the possibility that there is a very common depressive illness mainly affecting females and only occasionally males. This would explain the excess of female depressive patients in the families of bipolar subjects as a contaminant and would explain the high prevalence of females among the depressive subjects in the relatives of the control populations. In a sense, this suggests that a significant proportion of female depressive subjects who are found in families of bipolar patients could bear no genetic relationship at all to bipolar illness.

## Suicide Risks in Relatives of Schizophrenic, Manic, Depressive, and Control Subjects

Because the assessment of suicide risk is so important to clinicians, Tsuang (1983) assessed such risks in relatives of patient groups as well as control groups. The risk for suicide in relatives of schizophrenic, manic, and depressive subjects was 2.3%, which was eight times greater than the risk in relatives of control subjects. Relatives of patients (probands) who committed suicide were exposed to a 7.9% risk, which was four times higher than the 2.1% risk in the relatives of patients who did not commit suicide. The suicide risk of 1.2% in the relatives of schizophrenic subjects was close to the risk of 1.5% in the relatives of manic subjects, with the 3.4% risk of relatives of depression patients being significantly higher than that of the relatives of the schizophrenic or manic subjects. Nevertheless, the relatives of manic patients who had committed suicide showed an increased risk up to 9.4%, which was not significantly different from the 10.2% for the risk in relatives of depressive patients who committed suicide. In addition, the suicide risks in male relatives were higher than those in female relatives in all diagnostic categories. Interestingly, all of the suicides in relatives of schizophrenic patients occurred in males, suggesting that such relatives are particularly at risk. Most importantly, it would appear that the presence of a suicide in the proband increases the risk for suicide in an ill family member. Thus, 11.5% of deceased relatives of probands who themselves committed suicide died by suicide as opposed to only 3.7% of deceased relatives of probands who did not commit suicide. Whether this kind of association is related to a specific hereditary tendency to suicide, or similar environmental factors to which both proband and subject are exposed, is impossible to determine. Mitterauer (1990) evaluated epidemiologic data in five studies and noted that a predisposition to suicide is not necessarily the same genetic factor as found in endogenous psychoses. He suggested that psychological and social factors be considered equally with genetic factors. However, it is feasible that a propensity to suicide could be the outcome of two or more independently assorting genetic factors. One interesting possibility that lends itself to further investigation is that the affectively ill proband and his or her relatives entertain two independently assorting genetic factors, one for an affective illness and another for a specific type of personality that predisposes to suicide behavior. If these were found in the same person, that person when ill would be at a greater risk for suicide.

## Independent Familial Transmission of Psychotic Symptomatology

The above data on unipolar and bipolar illness suggest that the transmission of the illness is certainly familial and may well be genetic. Psychotic symptomatology (delusions and hallucinations), which is seen in a significant proportion of both unipolar and bipolar affective patients in the Iowa 500 study can be analyzed for the possibility of determining whether psychotic symptomatology was independently transmitted. To answer this, there were 22 usable pairs of proband-relative charts; all 22 relatives had been admitted to the same hospital (the Iowa Psychiatric Hospital) as had the bipolar and unipolar probands. Thus, each pair consisted of a proband and a family member, neither of whom had a diagnosis of schizophrenia. These pairs were evaluated as to whether or not both or neither member of the pair had psychotic symptoms or one member had such symptoms and the other did not. There was no evidence that psychotic symptoms bred true in this small study. Eleven pairs filled the psychosis positive/psychosis positive group or psychosis negative/psychosis negative group. The psychosis positive/psychosis negative groups also contained 11 pairs. For the data to support independent transmission of psychotic symptoms, it would have been necessary that the groups that were like for psychosis or like for the absence of psychosis be in the majority. This was not the case; in fact, the two groups were equal. Thus, though psychosis is a common phenomenon in both bipolar and unipolar affective disorder, it does not seem to be transmitted as a genetic variable (Winokur et al. 1986). What is responsible for psychotic symptomatology in the affective disorders is currently unknown.

## Familial Psychiatric Illness in Schizophrenia Versus Control Groups

The early family history material from our study (Winokur et al. 1972) suggested a familial factor in schizophrenia. Kendler and co-workers (1985b) evaluated this problem using DSM-III criteria. Of the original 200 schizophrenic patients in the Iowa 500 study, 173 met DSM-III criteria for schizophrenia. Of 310 schizophrenic patients (clinically diagnosed but did not meet research criteria) that were eliminated from the Iowa 500, 159 met criteria for schizophrenia consistent with the DSM-III criteria. For a group of control subjects, the original control subjects who had surgical procedures were supplemented by a set of control subjects for the nonselected clinically diagnosed schizophrenic subjects who did not meet the Feighner criteria originally. These control subjects were screened in order to eliminate any who had significant psychiatric illness or evidence of marked social maladjustment. Table 12–5 presents the material on the personally interviewed first-degree relatives of both schizophrenic patients and control patients. In the calculation of morbidity risks, the authors used varying ages at onset for the specific illnesses in the table. The statistical comparison in this table is based on the morbid risk findings, and it is clear that schizophrenia is more frequent in the family members of schizophrenic patients than in control subjects. Likewise, in this study schizoaffective disorder is more frequently seen in the families of schizophrenic patients than in the families of control subjects, and, when one adds up all of the nonaffective psychotic disorders, there is a very striking aggregation of these in the family background of the schizophrenic patients. Neither familial affective disorders nor anxiety disorders are different between the schizophrenic patients and control subjects, although alcoholism is seen more frequently in the family members of the control group.

In the table PCM is the prevalence corrected for mortality effects based on a total number of relatives who were interviewed or had a hospital record. Because there is an increased mortality in the disorders that are included in Table 12–5, if one did not correct for this, there would be a substantial underestimation of the true risk for disorders in relatives. By correcting for mortality, the disorders can be statistically compared without a confounding factor. The prevalence of schizophrenia in the interviewed relatives corrected for effects of differential mortality is probably the most accurate estimate of true risk. However, even here there may be some problem with underestimation; low fertility in schizophrenia as well as differential mobility may make these figures somewhat low. Nevertheless, there are striking differences in all nonaffective psychoses, as well as more rigorously defined schizophrenia, between the schizo-

**Table 12–5.** Morbid risks for psychiatric illness in primary interviewed relatives of schizophrenic and surgical control patients

| DSM-III-R disorder | Relatives of schizophrenic patients (N = 668) | | | | Relatives of Control patients (N = 1,043) | | | | |
|---|---|---|---|---|---|---|---|---|---|
| | N | Risk | MR ± SE | PCM | N | Risk | MR ± SE | PCM | P |
| Schizophrenia | 12 | 653 | 1.8 ± .5 | 2.7 | 0 | 919 | 0 | 0 | .0001 |
| Schizoaffective disorder | 5 | 520 | 1.0 ± .4 | 1.7 | 1 | 668 | .1 ± .1 | .1 | .5 |
| Paranoid disorder | 2 | 501 | .4 ± .3 | .5 | 0 | 507 | 0 | 0 | NS |
| Atypical psychosis | 4 | 520 | .8 ± .4 | .9 | 1 | 668 | .1 ± .1 | .1 | NS |
| All nonaffective psychotic disorder | 23 | 644 | 3.6 ± .7 | 5.3 | 2 | 889 | .2 ± .2 | .3 | .000001 |
| Unipolar illness | 32 | 586 | 5.5 ± .9 | 6.4 | 54 | 748 | 7.2 ± .9 | 6.7 | NS |
| Bipolar illness | 3 | 623 | .5 ± .3 | .6 | 3 | 851 | .4 ± .2 | .4 | NS |
| Anxiety disorder | 21 | 644 | 3.3 ± .7 | — | 41 | 889 | 4.6 ± .7 | — | NS |
| Alcoholism | 18 | 644 | 2.8 ± .6 | — | 17 | 889 | 5.3 ± .8 | — | .02 |

*Note.* MR ± SE = morbid risk ± standard error; PCM = prevalence corrected for mortality effects; NS = nonsignificant.
*Source.* Adapted from Kendler et al. 1985a.

phrenic families and the control families. Kendler and co-workers (1985b) present an interesting comparison related to these findings. They calculated a correlation of liability for schizophrenia and other disorders in first-degree relatives. This correlation varies between a relatively high .37 and .43, which suggests that familial factors play a significant role in transmission of schizophrenia. They put this figure into perspective by comparing it with the correlation of liability of first-degree relatives for other medical conditions in which familial genetic factors are thought to play an etiologic role: for pyloric stenosis, .40; for clubfoot, .35; for ischemic heart disease, .33; for diabetes mellitus, .27–.40; for peptic ulcer disease, .18–.27; and for hypertension, .24. Though such a familial comparison as this does not prove a genetic factor in schizophrenia, it is in favor of such a possibility when one takes into account that adoption studies have clearly supported an unequivocal genetic etiology for schizophrenia (Kety 1983; Kety et al. 1975).

## Subtypes in Schizophrenia

The question of whether there is a familial difference between paranoid schizophrenia and nonparanoid (hebephrenic-catatonic) schizophrenia remains a matter of extreme importance, both for research and clinical purposes. Kendler and colleagues (1988) evaluated paranoid and nonparanoid schizophrenia classified according to Tsuang and Winokur (1974) criteria by analyzing DSM-III criteria in first-degree relatives of schizophrenic probands. In addition to the Tsuang and Winokur criteria, the authors used other diagnostic systems to subdivide schizophrenia into paranoid and nonparanoid subtypes.

The results showed no significant difference in risk for either schizophrenia alone or for nonaffective psychotic disorders in the relatives as a function of the subtype diagnosis. The subtypes were paranoid, hebephrenic, catatonic, and undifferentiated, and the numbers of probands were, respectively, 68,

50, 13, and 121. Also, no significant difference was found in the risk for affective disorders in the relatives of these schizophrenic probands by subtype. Specifically, separating probands according to Tsuang and Winokur criteria into paranoid, hebephrenic, and an undetermined subtype, they found in the paranoid patients a familial morbid risk for affective disorder of 6.9%; for the hebephrenic patients, it was 2.6%; and for the undetermined subtype, it was 3.3%.

Although previous studies have sometimes found evidence for significant subtype resemblance in pairs of affected relatives, concordance for subtype never exceeded chance expectation. In general, the result of the investigation suggested that familial factors affect the person's liability to schizophrenia but do not greatly influence specific subtypes. Interestingly, however, the agreement in subtype diagnosis between schizophrenic probands and their schizophrenic relatives using the Tsuang and Winokur criteria and ICD-9 criteria showed concordances of 45.8% and 52.6%, respectively, which, while not significant, suggest some value in further study.

Kendler and Tsuang (1988) also evaluated outcome and familial psychopathology in schizophrenia, and they found no relationship between any dimension of outcome in schizophrenic patients and amount of risk in their relatives for schizophrenia. There was also no relationship between proband outcome and familial risk for all nonaffective psychoses. When subtyping schizophrenia, paranoid schizophrenic subjects did better than nonparanoid schizophrenic subjects in terms of outcome. On the other hand, in the study of subtypes by Kendler and colleagues (1988), there was no increase in risk for schizophrenia in any of the subtypes. Putting these two findings together, one would certainly have predicted no relationship between amount of familial psychopathology and outcome, which is not surprising.

The data from the Iowa 500 study were used to test various models of transmission of schizophrenia. Tsuang and co-workers (1982) used the data to employ a segregation analysis in order to determine if transmission of schizophrenia could be explained by a single major gene. The results suggested that a monogenic hypothesis could not account for the transmission of schizophrenia, meaning both a recessive and a dominant transmission theory were rejected. There was evidence of parent-child transmission, and this could have been either psychosocial in cause or an interaction between genetic and psychosocial factors. The authors point out that a genetic heterogeneity is likely in the sample and that several different illnesses could be masquerading under the same clinical diagnosis or symptomatology. Heterogeneity in the group of schizophrenic subjects of the Iowa 500 makes it very difficult, if not impossible, to evaluate the type of transmission in a meaningful manner.

Tsuang and colleagues (1983a) also used this data to evaluate the problem of schizophrenia spectrum disorders. Using a multiple threshold model and applying it to the blind family study data, they found that the proportion of relatives receiving any psychiatric diagnosis other than schizophrenia and affective disorder was the same between the families of schizophrenic and control probands, meaning the data did not fit the model. They were unable to accept the hypothesis that schizophrenia, as a spectrum of disorders defined according to standard diagnostic nomenclature, had a common familial etiology. The spectrum that was investigated included neuroses, personality disorders, and other nonorganic psychoses. As suggested by other studies, one could have included personality disorders such as schizotypal personality disorder and paranoid personality disorder in the spectrum that includes schizophrenia (Baron et al. 1985).

The question of sex differences in the familial transmission of schizophrenia in the Iowa 500 sample was evaluated by Goldstein and co-workers (1990). The lifetime morbidity risks of schizophrenia for relatives of male schizophrenic probands was 2.2% but was considerably higher—5.2%—for relatives of female schizophrenic probands ($P = .047$). The difference in familial morbidity risks for the sexes also remained when the definition of illness in probands included both schizophreniform and schizoaffective disorders. For all three disorders, it was 3.6% in relatives of male probands versus 6.3% in relatives of female probands ($P = .09$). In siblings alone, there is an even larger difference—for males, 2.8%; for females, 7.9% ($P = .03$). However, sex differences between male and female relatives with schizophrenia or spectrum disorders showed no significant differences; for male relatives, the risk for schizophrenia plus spectrum disorders was 10.4% and for female relatives, 8.1% (not significant). Likewise, as predicted from these data, there was no concordance between sex of proband and sex of affected sibling. There was significantly higher risk for schizotypal personality among relatives of male schizophrenic patients compared with relatives of female schizophrenic patients. If schizophrenia were transmitted by many genes rather than one gene and a male required fewer genes for the illness to express itself, he would be predicted to have fewer relatives with the same illness or might have relatives with a mild form of the illness. However, at this point it is not possible to explain clearly the reason for the differences, and more sophisticated genetic studies need to be performed.

# Chapter 13

# Early Clinical and Family History Findings in Light of the Final Feighner Diagnosis

*Admission Clinical Picture and Family History Relevant to Follow-Up Diagnosis*

It may seem like gilding the lily to write a chapter such as this, but hindsight is better than foresight in this case.

We have already discussed the early clinical findings using the systematic diagnosis made from the charts. However, few other studies exist where those findings may be reexamined in the light of the final diagnosis, which is made on the basis of a period of observation spanning 30–40 years after the index admission.

The model is clearly that of Kahlbaum and Kraepelin in the late 1800s, when these earlier psychiatrists took into account both the clinical picture and the course of the illness. However, they did not have a systematic set of operational criteria with which to choose people. Instead, they used their clinical material to make sensible diagnoses. Modern studies indicate that it is possible to make reliable and valid diagnoses using systematic research criteria. Therefore, we now present the clinical background, the early course of the illness, and the family history in light of the final diagnoses. We started by making a diagnosis according to the research criteria and ended 30–40 years later by making a diagnosis according to the same criteria. We have already looked at the end states of the patients after a long follow-up in previous chapters. Here we will examine the circumstances that surround the index admission by a few years.

To accomplish this, we needed a set of reasonable research criteria, and the only diagnostic system that was available at the time the study was started was that of the Feighner et al. criteria (1972). These have also been termed the St. Louis criteria or the Washington University criteria because it was at Washington University in St. Louis where the criteria were first formulated. Specific criteria had already been published at the time by Cassidy and co-workers (1957) on depression, by Purtell and colleagues (1951) on hysteria, and by Wheeler and associates (1950) on anxiety neurosis. The criteria of Cassidy and co-workers for depression were essentially as follows: the patient made a statement of mood change (e.g., blue or discouraged) and had 6 of 10 symptoms that were slow thinking, anorexia, constipation, insomnia, fatigue, loss of concentration, suicidal ideas, weight loss, decreased sex interest, agitation, and marked complaining, or, in the best judgment of the examiner, the correct diagnosis was manic depressive disease. Certainly, these have much in common with the Feighner criteria and may well have been equally as reliable. After the Feighner criteria, there were several new series of sets of criteria, namely the Research Diagnostic Criteria (RDC), DSM-III, and DSM-III-R. There is a large overlap between these and the Feighner criteria although they are not identical. No doubt they, too, could have been used for a reliable study of some of the characteristics of the illnesses that were involved. In fact, Kendler and colleagues (1985b) used the DSM-III criteria for a family study of psychiatric illness in first-degree relatives of schizophrenic versus surgical control patients. In this study of schizophrenia, the DSM-III diagnoses were made from the index chart only. They found that the DSM-III criteria were quite useful in separating patients in order to determine the specificities of family backgrounds in schizophrenic versus control subjects. Coryell and Zimmerman (1987) compared different sets of criteria (i.e., Feighner, RDC, and DSM-III) and found few reasons to believe that one was superior to the other. They subjected the criteria to a short follow-up and an examination of familial psychiatric illness as validators and noted that all three sets of criteria were useful in separating different diagnoses. However, this study did not have the benefit of a very long follow-up and the assessment of patients who had a stable diagnosis. Consequently, we believe there is place for an assessment of the clinical background of a set of patients in whom the diagnoses were validated by a long follow-up that considered both the clinical background and the outcome in terms of the change in diagnosis, if warranted.

## The Stability of Diagnosis

Not all patients had the kind of follow-up that made it possible to make reasonable final diagnoses. Thus, there is a decrease in the number of patients from the original 525 first selected. Some patients became undiagnosed, which lowered the number of bipolar, depressive, and schizophrenic patients who could be evaluated. The following data on diagnostic stability are based on the same set of diagnostic criteria (Feighner) for index assessment and for the diagnosis that was made in light of a long follow-up.

Of 143 unipolar patients (originally diagnosed according to the Feighner criteria), who had final diagnoses after 30–40 years, 5 (4%) became schizophrenic, and 4 of 5 became hebephrenic-catatonic in nature. On the other hand, 19 of the unipolar patients became undiagnosed; thus, the person evaluating these records and follow-ups was not certain that it was possible to diagnose them as unipolar depressive.

Of 66 original bipolar patients who had a high-quality follow-up, 4 became schizophrenic (all hebephrenic-catatonic), and 9 of the 66 (14%) of the bipolar patients became undiagnosed. It was possible to reconstitute the group of bipolar patients by adding the 22 unipolar patients who had become bipolar in time, which left us with 88 bipolar patients of whom 11 (13%) became undiagnosed. It is interesting to note this final bipolar group included three originally diagnosed as schizophrenic. When all of the data were finally evaluated, we found that 23 (16%) of the 146 originally diagnosed unipolar patients (who appeared in the final sample) had become manic. If one uses the base number of 225 that were originally diagnosed as unipolar, the 23 patients who changed show a 10.2% proportion of unipolar patients who will change over time. Of the original 211 affective disorder patients (in whom there was good long-term follow-up), 30 (14%) were considered undiagnosed in follow-up, and 9 (4%) had a final diagnosis of schizophrenia.

Of 170 schizophrenic patients (both hebephrenic-catatonic and paranoid), one became unipolar after the long follow-up, which was less than 1%. There were 3 of the 170 who became bipolar (2%), and of the 170 schizophrenic patients, 8 (5%) became undiagnosed. Thus, there are data on 170 schizophrenic at time of index, 66 bipolar at time of index, 23 depressive who became manic at time of index, and 123 unipolar subjects. The final diagnoses in the long-term follow-up according to the Feighner criteria included 98 unipolar, 79 bipolar, 122 hebephrenic-catatonic schizophrenic, 45 paranoid schizophrenic, and 38 undiagnosed patients. These diagnoses reflect information that was gleaned at index by follow-up exams, by medical records, and by information from letters and other communication from relatives, physicians, and social agencies.

## Clinical Symptomatology

As expected, the final Feighner diagnoses reflected the criteria that were originally used to select patients. The unipolar depressive subjects had the largest number of depressive symptoms, the bipolar subjects mainly admitted for mania had large numbers of manic symptoms, and the schizophrenic subjects were the main possessors of the schizophrenic symptoms. Some other findings were interesting: as a group, the patients who were undiagnosed had many depressive symptoms at index admission, with records showing 63% had dysphoria, 63% had anorexia, 84% had sleep difficulty, 61% had trouble concentrating, 18% had made suicide attempts, and 24% had suicide thoughts. The latter two symptoms had been seen frequently in only the unipolar depressive group. Some of the finally undiagnosed patients had euphoria (29%), hyperactivity (26%), and pressure of speech (26%). Some of the undiagnosed patients also had some schizophrenic-type symptoms, including altered perception, which was seen in 26% as opposed to only 7% and 8% of the affective disorder patients. They were also more likely to have persecutory delusions (71%) and auditory hallucinations (32%). There was a reason, therefore, for the undiagnosed follow-up to be considered under that rubric because they had a large admixture of symptoms from other groups. It is noteworthy that not only did the undiagnosed include those patients who were difficult to diagnose as affective or schizophrenic but also included a certain number who were difficult to diagnose as hebephrenic-catatonic or paranoid. They are a very mixed group, and, as they are constituted, it is unlikely that we can learn very much from them.

The more soluble problem is how many of the schizophrenic and affective disorder patients shared specific depressive, manic, and schizophrenic symptoms. Though the unipolar depressive patients had 94% sleep difficulty (all types) and 89% of the bipolar patients had sleep difficulty, 39% of the hebephrenic-catatonic patients and 27% of the paranoid patients had this symptom. Loss of energy was more frequently seen in depressive patients (73%), but it was also seen in 18%–25% of the schizophrenic patients. Loss of interest was seen in 91% of the unipolar, and in 57 (40%) of the schizophrenic patients. Sexual drive was decreased equally in unipolar, hebephrenic, and paranoid patients (24%–31%). Problems in concentration were seen in 55% of the unipolar patients but also in 33%–36% of the schizophrenic patients. Thus, there is a fair amount of overlap between the symptoms of depression both in schizophrenia and in unipolar depression in particular. The symptoms of mania were much more specific to the bipolar group but distractibility, which was seen in 67% of bipolar patients, was seen in 43% of hebephrenic-catatonic patients and 31% of paranoid schizophrenic patients.

Regarding schizophrenic-type symptoms, there was also overlap. Delusions of depersonalization and derealization were seen in 16% of all the schizophrenic but in 13% of the unipolar depressive subjects. Persecutory delusions were seen in 49%–52% of the affective disorder patients and in 84%–100% of the schizophrenic subjects, with the overlap being obviously very large. It is clear that the symptom pictures as presented in the Feighner criteria are useful as a group, but some symptoms are less discriminatory than others.

Table 13–1 shows a systematic evaluation of the resolving power of the symptoms of mania when the bipolar and the schizophrenic patients are compared. This is presented in terms of an odds ratio (OR), the formula being

$$OR = \frac{A \times D}{B \times C}$$

The odds of having a manic symptom in the bipolar group = A/B. The odds of having a manic symptom in the chronic nonaffective psychosis (CNAP) group = C/D. For euphoria and/or irritability (Table 13–1) the formula is

$$OR = \frac{53 \times 161}{26 \times 6} = 54.7$$

The ORs present approximates risks for symptoms among the diagnostic groups.

The numerator in the first column and second column (Table 13–1) is the number of probands who showed that particular symptom; the denominator is those who lacked that symptom. The OR is an assessment of the strength of the symptom in separating the groups; the larger the ratio, the stronger the resolving

**Table 13–1.** Resolving power of symptoms of mania and schizophrenia symptoms in a comparison of patients with mania with chronic nonaffective psychosis

| | Bipolar $N = 79$ | CNAP $N = 167$ | OR |
|---|---|---|---|
| **Mania symptoms** | Present/ absent | Present/ absent | |
| Euphoria and/ or irritability | 53/26 | 6/161 | 54.7 |
| Hyperactivity | 55/24 | 10/151 | 34.6 |
| Pressure of speech | 52/27 | 8/159 | 38.3 |
| Flight of ideas | 46/33 | 4/163 | 56.8 |
| Grandiosity (delusional) | 10/69 | 19/148 | 1.12 |
| Grandiosity (other) | 14/65 | 6/161 | 5.8 |
| Distractibility | 53/26 | 67/100 | 3 |
| Excessive spending | 10/69 | 3/164 | 7.9 |
| Sleep difficulty | 70/9 | 59/108 | 14.2 |
| Agitation | 43/36 | 39/128 | 3.9 |
| **Schizophrenia symptoms** | | | |
| Poor premorbid adjustment | 5/74 | 83/84 | 14.6 |
| Passivity delusions | 2/77 | 66/101 | 25.2 |
| Depersonalization/ derealization | 4/75 | 27/140 | 3.6 |
| Changed perception | 6/73 | 44/123 | 4.4 |
| Symbolism | 1/78 | 45/122 | 28.8 |
| Persecutory delusions | 39/40 | 147/20 | 2.4 |
| Auditory hallucinations | 11/68 | 87/80 | 6.7 |
| Visual hallucinations | 5/74 | 45/122 | 5.5 |
| Haptic hallucinations | 3/76 | 46/121 | 9.6 |
| Blocking, mute, tangential | 4/75 | 97/70 | 30 |
| Motor symptoms | 7/72 | 54/113 | 4.9 |
| Flat, inappropriate affect | 2/77 | 117/50 | 90.1 |

*Note.* CNAP = chronic nonaffective psychosis; OR = odds ratio.

power. Euphoria and flight of ideas are extremely discriminating, but distractibility is poorly discriminating as is delusional grandiosity. Although there have been a series of new sets of diagnostic criteria, there is still a place for an investigation of discriminating power of each symptom that is used in these criteria sets. Clearly, not all symptoms are equally discriminating (Table 13–1). Some are more useful than others, and perhaps it would be possible to make diagnostic criteria that essentially use the symptoms and characteristics that were noted to produce high OR for mania and chronic nonaffective psychoses, mainly schizophrenia. Table 13–2 shows OR comparing the patients with unipolar depression and those with chronic nonaffective psychoses. As with the comparison with manic patients, there is a range of magnitudes in OR, but they are not as striking as in the comparisons between mania and schizophrenia.

## Noncriterion Items

Symptoms such as anxiety attacks, many somatic complaints, phobias, obsessional thinking, and compulsive behavior did not discriminate the groups. One to 3% of the groups showed anxiety attacks, 1%–2% of the groups showed phobias, and 3%–4% showed obsessions and compulsions. Somatic complaints were seen most frequently in paranoid schizophrenic patients (13%), next in hebephrenic-catatonic patients (8%), and in 3%–4% of the affective disorder patients. Organic symptoms picked up by mental status showed no significant difference. Eight to 13% of the affective disorder patients showed memory deficits, whereas 2%–18% of the schizophrenic patients showed such symptoms. Some of the symptoms that did discriminate the groups are presented in Table 13–3. Antisocial behavior, though not significantly different by a $2 \times K$ chi-square analysis, is obviously more frequent in the schizophrenic groups than in the affective disorder groups.

## Preadmission Course of Illness and Short-Term Follow-Up

The majority of the patients in this study were first-admission patients. They were generally well educated, which can be seen in the hebephrenic-catatonic patients where 66% had gone to high school or further; the same proportion of the bipolar patients also had this similar educational experience. The unipo-

**Table 13–2.** Resolving power of symptoms of depression and schizophrenia in a comparison of patients with unipolar depression and chronic nonaffective psychosis

|  | Unipolar $N = 98$ | CNAP $N = 167$ | OR |
|---|---|---|---|
| **Depression symptoms** | Present/ absent | Present/ absent |  |
| Length 3 months or less at index | 43/55 | 5/162 | 23.3 |
| Retardation | 62/36 | 13/154 | 20.4 |
| Self-reproach | 72/26 | 14/153 | 30.3 |
| Diurnal variation | 18/80 | 1/166 | 37.35 |
| Anorexia | 77/21 | 29/138 | 17.4 |
| Weight loss | 38/60 | 15/152 | 6.4 |
| Loss of interest | 89/9 | 88/79 | 8.8 |
| **Schizophrenia symptoms** |  |  |  |
| Poor premorbid adjustment | 2/96 | 83/84 | 47.4 |
| Passivity delusions | 2/96 | 66/101 | 31.3 |
| Depersonalization/ realization | 13/85 | 27/140 | 1.3 |
| Changed perception | 7/91 | 44/123 | 4.7 |
| Persecutory delusions | 51/47 | 147/20 | 6.8 |
| Auditory hallucinations | 7/91 | 87/80 | 14.1 |
| Haptic hallucinations | 7/91 | 46/121 | 4.9 |
| Blocking, mute, tangential | 4/94 | 97/70 | 32.6 |
| Flat, inappropriate affect | 1/97 | 117/50 | 226.98 |

*Note.* CNAP = chronic nonaffective psychosis; OR = odds ratio; nonaffective psychoses = hebephrenic-catatonic and paranoid schizophrenia, delusional disorder.

**Table 13–3.** Noncriteria symptoms according to clinical groups

| Symptoms | Unipolar N = 98 | Bipolar N = 79 | Hebephrenic-catatonic N = 122 | Paranoid schizophrenic N = 45 | Undiagnosed N = 38 | P |
|---|---|---|---|---|---|---|
| Loss of interest | 89 (91) | 27 (34) | 70 (57) | 18 (40) | 21 (55) | .0001 |
| Sex drive, decreased | 25 (26) | 10 (13) | 29 (24) | 14 (31) | 5 (13) | .0001 |
| Sex drive, increased | 2 (2) | 21 (27) | 14 (11) | 5 (11) | 4 (11) | .0001 |
| Increased tearfulness | 62 (63) | 32 (41) | 29 (24) | 8 (18) | 19 (50) | .0001 |
| Diurnal variation | 18 (18) | 7 (9) | 1 (<1) | 0 (0) | 3 (8) | .0001 |
| Antisocial behavior | 1 (1) | 2 (3) | 8 (7) | 4 (9) | 1 (3) | .116 |

*Note.*   Values are *n* (%).

lar depressive and the paranoid schizophrenic groups were high school graduates or better in 43%–51% of the cases, respectively. These were the older patients in the study, and it is likely that opportunities for that much education were not available so freely to these patients. Table 13–4 gives a variety of other preindex characteristics. As shown in the table, acute onset, defined as the time from onset of illness to time of index hospitalization, is much shorter for the affective disorder patients than for the schizophrenic patients. Between the unipolar and bipolar patients, the acuteness was far more clear in the bipolar patients, who were three times more likely to have had two or more prior admissions. The schizophrenic patients are far more likely to have never been married. The unipolar depressive patients are somewhat more likely to have had precipitating factors in their background that include psychosocial factors as well as medical and biological difficulties.

Most interesting is that, unknowingly, the clinicians at the University of Iowa Psychiatric Hospital were very likely to diagnose the patients in accordance with systematic criteria. Thus, 95% of the unipolar patients had an affective disorder diagnosis, which conforms to the Feighner criteria, as did 88% of the bipolar patients. Most of the schizophrenic patients diagnosed by research criteria had a diagnosis of schizophrenia by the clinicians. The final undiagnosed group has a fairly sizable admixture of clinical diagnoses because it not only includes patients who were undiagnosed as to whether they had an affective illness or a schizophrenic illness, but also a certain number of patients in whom it was impossible to determine whether they were hebephrenic-catatonic or paranoid. The patients were diagnosed according to whether they had had prior episodes as well as prior psychiatric hospital admissions. It is clear that if these are reliable data, episodes are often not likely to lead to hospitalization. There are more affective disorder patients who experience their first admission than who experience their first episode. In other words, they had undergone prior episodes that had not necessitated hospitalization. Thirteen percent of the unipolar depressive patients had experienced two or more prior

**Table 13–4.** Preindex variables and hospital course according to clinical groups

| | Unipolar N = 98 | Bipolar N = 79 | Hebephrenic-catatonic N = 122 | Paranoid schizophrenic N = 45 | Undiagnosed N = 38 | P |
|---|---|---|---|---|---|---|
| Age at admission median years | 41 | 33 | 26 | 35 | 27 | .0001 |
| Age at onset, median years | 39 | 27 | 22 | 29 | 26 | .0002 |
| Never married | 17 (17) | 31 (39) | 95 (78) | 25 (56) | 13 (34) | .0001 |
| Precipitating factors, none | 54 (54) | 56 (71) | 105 (86) | 42 (93) | 29 (76) | .0001 |
| Length of illness prior to hospital admission: | | | | | | |
| 3 months or less | 43 (34) | 56 (71) | 3 (2) | 2 (4) | 16 (42) | .0001 |
| 3 years or more | 4 (4) | 2 (3) | 48 (39) | 30 (67) | 5 (13) | .0001 |
| Index episode first episode | 56 (57) | 38 (48) | 111 (91) | 45 (100) | 30 (79) | .0001 |
| One or more prior episodes | 42 (43) | 41 (52) | 11 (8) | 0 (0) | 8 (21) | .0001 |
| Index admit, first admit | 81 (83) | 50 (63) | 92 (75) | 36 (80) | 32 (84) | NS |
| Two or more prior admits | 5 (5) | 13 (16) | 10 (8) | 3 (7) | 2 (5) | NS |
| Discharged to community | 32 (33) | 29 (37) | 24 (20) | 6 (13) | 17 (35) | .006 |
| Hospital diagnosis | | | | | | |
| Affective disorder | (95) | (88) | (4) | (4) | (71) | |
| Schizophrenia | (1) | (4) | (93) | (80) | (24) | |
| Other | (4) | | | | | |

Note   Values are *n* (5).

episodes, but only 5% had experienced two or more prior admissions. On the other hand, the schizophrenic patients had more prior admissions than prior episodes, indicating that they had been chronically ill and were hospitalized for essentially the same episode on more than one occasion.

Table 13–5 gives the results of the short-term follow-up. For all the groups together, only 6% had no follow-up. Seventy-four percent of the follow-up was by letters and the remainder by other means such as readmissions to hospital, admissions to state hospital, contacts with relatives by social workers and doctors, and so forth. Neither the hebephrenic patients nor the paranoid schizophrenic patients were likely to have had a complete recovery at any point during the short-term follow-up. In fact, the hebephrenic-catatonic patients had the longest follow-up of any, and they had the least amount of total remission.

If one adds those patients with a complete recovery at some point, those with a social recovery, and those outside the hospital or possibly socially recovered, 64% of the unipolar patients fit these categories, 77% of the bipolar patients, 17% of the hebephrenic-catatonic schizophrenic patients, and 20% of the paranoid schizophrenic patients. For the undiagnosed subjects, these categories of improvement (not necessarily total recovery) encompassed 63%. Interestingly, the undiagnosed group had made a complete recovery in 47% of the cases, making them at least in follow-up very similar to the affective disorder patients. Regarding one or more subsequent admissions to the University of Iowa Psychiatric Hospital, it was clear that the largest contributors to this were the bipolar patients, of whom 22% were readmitted to the same hospital for another episode versus 8%–11% of the other groups.

## Family History of Psychiatric Illness

Table 13–6 presents the family history of schizophrenia, affective disorder, alcoholism, and minor psychiatric illness in the unipolar, bipolar, and schizophrenic patients. Schizophrenia is

**Table 13–5.**　Short-term follow-up according to final systematic diagnosis of clinical groups

|  | Unipolar N = 98 | Bipolar N = 79 | Hebephrenic-catatonic N = 122 | Paranoid schizophrenic N = 45 | Undiagnosed N = 38 | P |
|---|---|---|---|---|---|---|
| No short-term follow-up, n (%) | 6 (6) | 6 (8) | 7 (6) | 2 (4) | 2 (5) | |
| Length, follow-up, years | 3.8 | 3.0 | 4.8 | 2.0 | 3.4 | |
| One or more subsequent admits, n (%) | 10 (10) | 17 (22) | 10 (8) | 5 (11) | 3 (8) | .02 |
| Complete recovery at some point, % | 45 | 45 | 47 | 4.9 | 6.7 | .05 |
| Social recovery, not complete, % | 8.2 | 7.6 | 6.6 | 4.4 | 53 | 47 |
| Never well, socially unrecovered or deteriorated, % | 30 | 14 | 77 | 76 | 32 | |
| Uncertain, but social recovery or outside the hospital, % | 11 | 22 | 5.7 | 8.0 | 11 | |

**Table 13-6.** Comparison of the family history (parents and siblings) in unipolar, bipolar, and schizophrenic patients

| | Unipolar $N = 98$ | | | | Bipolar $N = 79$ | | | | Schizophrenic $N = 165$ | | | |
|---|---|---|---|---|---|---|---|---|---|---|---|---|
| | Family (n) | Family at risk | Ill | Morbid risk (%) | Family (n) | Family at risk | Ill | Morbid risk (%) | Family (n) | Family at risk | Ill | Morbid risk (%) |
| Schizophrenia | 634 | 519 | 4 | .77 | 434 | 398 | 2 | .50 | 851 | 763 | 12 | 1.57 |
| Affective disorder | 634 | 468 | 54 | 11.5 | 434 | 235 | 28 | 11.9 | 851 | 429 | 20 | 4.7 |
| Alcoholism[a] | 319 | 262 | 12 | 4.6 | 224 | 211 | 16 | 7.6 | 410 | 374 | 25 | 6.7 |
| Minor psychiatric illness[b] | 185 | 185 | 16 | 8.6 | 146 | 146 | 25 | 17.1 | 320 | 320 | 67 | 20.9 |

*Note.* Risk period: schizophrenia, 20–40; affective disorder, 20–60; alcoholism, 20–40.
[a]Males.
[b]Parents only, all at risk if information was available.

relatively uncommon in the first-degree relatives but is seen two to three times more frequently in the schizophrenic families than in the affective disorder families. Affective disorder, comprising mania and depression, is seen 2.5 times more frequently in the families of the affective disorder probands. Alcoholism does not appear to differentiate the groups, but it is of some interest that minor psychiatric illnesses (neuroses, personality disorders) are seen less than half as frequently in the relatives of the unipolar depressive group than in the other two groups. For the affective disorder probands taken together, 12% of the parents had minor psychiatric illnesses; this was found in almost twice as many parents (21%) of the schizophrenic probands.

An assessment was made of psychiatric illness on the maternal and/or paternal sides of the families. In the bipolar and unipolar subjects, 20.3% had an affective disorder in the more distant relatives. In the schizophrenic patients, 16% had affective disorder on the maternal and paternal sides. Thus, there is an increase of 25% in the distant relatives of the affective disorder patients. For schizophrenia, the finding is more striking. Five of 177 patients with affective disorder had schizophrenia on one side of the family, but of 167 schizophrenic patients, this was seen for 12 of the probands. Though the numbers are small, the difference is between 3% and 7%, which is of course over double in the families of schizophrenic patients. There were no obvious differences between maternal and paternal sides of the family for any of these illnesses. Alcoholism was seen in 7%–8% of the extended families of the affective disorder patients but in 16% of the extended families of the schizophrenic patients. In general, alcoholism was more frequently seen on the paternal side of the families of the probands where 29 of the paternal sides contained alcoholism as opposed to 16 of the maternal sides.

The findings of the family history analyses are similar to those findings for the entire group when it was not corrected for change in diagnosis. Essentially this suggests that the diagnosis that was made by the Feighner criteria predicts family history. Presumably, similar operational criteria sets will be useful in assignment to groups for research as well as for treatment.

# Chapter 14

# Zero-Symptom Schizophrenia

*Symptoms Present in Schizophrenic*
*Patients After a 30- to 40-Year Follow-Up*

Some investigators have noted in follow-up that some schizophrenic patients have a good outcome. (Bleuler 1978; Chiompi 1980; Harding et al. 1987; Johnstone et al. 1984). Perhaps the most impressive data are those of Johnstone and co-workers who identified a series of schizophrenic patients using the Feighner research criteria and followed up 66 of them after 5–9 years. They found that 18% of the patients had no significant symptoms and appeared to function satisfactorily, and, of the 12 patients who had recovered, 11 were female.

This is a somewhat more optimistic outcome than was found by McCreadie (1982). Of 133 schizophrenic patients in an English community, 97 were positive for the Feighner criteria. At the Creighton Royal Hospital, all were inpatients or outpatients who had a diagnosis of schizophrenia; thus, all were in psychiatric care at the time that they were evaluated. Eighteen percent had no abnormalities in their mental status, and 21% had no abnormalities of behavior. However, only 3% had no abnormalities in either mental status or behavior. It should be noted that, as all of the patients were in treatment at the hospital either as outpatients or inpatients, it is unlikely that those who had recovered were included in the sample.

Such studies as the above are rather unusual with the more common kind of assessment typified by a study of Johnstone and co-workers (1985, 1990), in which first-episode schizophrenic patients were followed for a period of 2 years. Poor outcome was associated with more social withdrawal, inactivity, and abnormal social presentation as well as with more "neurological soft signs." A good occupational outcome in patients was associated with a short duration of illness prior to treatment, and, surprisingly, in the patients with a short pretreatment duration of illness, a good occupational outcome was associated with placebo medication during the follow-up. The fact that a shorter duration was associated with a better outcome is not surprising in that many studies (Stephens et al. 1960; Valliant 1964) suggest that acuteness of onset is associated with a good prognosis. However, in those good prognosis patients, the fact that prescription of placebo rather than medication was associated with a good occupational outcome deserves more study, as was noted by the authors themselves. But the fact happens to be that in this extremely useful study, it is not possible to determine how many of the patients were absolutely, unequivocally well at the time of the follow-up or how many had achieved that status in the 2 years prior to being reevaluated. Thus, the Johnstone et al. 1990 study is more typical of the literature, but the Johnstone et al. 1984 study comes closer to answering questions as to how many patients are, in fact, well at the time of follow-up.

The Iowa 500 gives us the opportunity to evaluate patients after a long period of follow-up and specifically gives us the opportunity to determine both their mental status and behavior 30–40 years after index admission as well as to evaluate the subjects' symptoms present at follow-up. The fact that a large group of these index schizophrenic patients were systematically interviewed at follow-up and the fact that we were able to get good mental hospital records give us an unusual opportunity to examine the course of schizophrenia over the long haul. This is a particularly important point in that it bears directly on Bleuler's (1978) observation that a large number of schizophrenic patients could be considered recovered. Bleuler, of course, had the opportunity to interact personally with patients over many years. However, he adopted a rather wide latitude in what he considered recovery in that he said, "Probands were also considered recovered when a thorough medical examination uncovered some residues of delusional ideas, faulty perception relative to their former psychosis, eccentricity or constriction in their fields of interest or activity." Thus, Bleuler's own observations suggested the schizophrenic patients were improved but not totally recovered.

Bleuler, in the tradition of all accomplished clinicians, presented some accounts of his recovered schizophrenic patients. One of his patients (EZ) was born in 1912 and became schizophrenic around 1929. Then, around 1961, she began to improve and became more communicative, more coherent in her thinking, less delusional, and less hallucinatory. However, by around the age of 50, she developed memory deficits. In 1967, at 55, she was suffering from a markedly impaired memory but no longer said anything about delusions or hallucinations and was considered a kind and friendly person. She regarded her hospitalization as acceptable and showed no desire to leave the clinic. It is interesting in the case of EZ that she no longer said anything about delusions or hallucinations, but it is entirely possible that she still entertained them, though they no longer had much force that would lead to expression. Additionally, her memory difficulties and her lack of interest in leaving the hospital make one suspect that she was perhaps still affected by schizophrenia.

Another interesting case is that of ES, who was born in 1912 and at age 31, in 1943, was admitted to the clinic. Twenty years later, in 1963, a period of improvement set in. He began to take an interest in things and read newspapers, and his family no longer regarded him as mentally ill but simply as somewhat odd.

However, he still had delusional associations and led a somewhat isolated life limited to the confines of his family.

In the case of JZ, born in 1910, schizophrenia manifested itself at age 29 in 1938, but in 1958 a slight improvement was noted and progressed further. Ultimately, he entered a home for the unemployable and got along well with his housemates who considered him to be a likable person. Bleuler himself evaluated JZ and found him interested as well as warmly and genuinely pleased to meet Bleuler again. However, when JZ was questioned about his former delusions, he still held to them and responded to such questions in a confused and distracted manner similar to before.

RR was born in 1900 and became ill in 1925 when he was diagnosed as having schizophrenia with delusions of grandeur and persecution. In 1936, he was in a state of "manic-hebephrenic excitation" but quieted down, improved, and was released after 6 months. He was in good shape for about 4 years, and then had a renewed onset of excitation in 1942 when he destroyed furniture and shrubbery in the garden, which necessitated a third hospitalization. He had several long undisturbed years with many productive periods of employment but was rehospitalized in 1950. After 15 months, he was again released and, since that time, has required no further hospitalization. This patient appears to have had rather acute onset with multiple episodes, and one might question the possibility that he suffered from an affective disorder (manic-depressive illness) rather than schizophrenia. The course of the illness may be as good a characteristic of a psychiatric disease as the phenomenology.

EG was born 1898 and became ill around age 23. He was followed to age 66 and still seemed somewhat monotonous and flat, holding to unusual philosophical convictions that were hard to follow. He also had unusual body sensations and felt "vibrations" in his body. He said that he must purge "blasphemous thoughts" that came to him with his religious thoughts. Bleuler considered him a bit odd and eccentric but not mentally ill.

Finally, there was the case of CE, born in 1890. She was obviously psychotic and, in 1940, Bleuler himself evaluated the patient and noted that she was well groomed with no psychotic symptoms in evidence. However, she had zero insight into her own previously severe psychosis, and, when confronted with the symptoms, she disputed their existence and made light of them. She was happy with her treatment at the psychiatric hospital and had no initiative to reshape her life into becoming useful and independent. Her schizophrenia became chronic at 49. It is notable that although she had no more new schizophrenic symptoms, she lost initiative for normal life and had no insight into the illness.

These case studies are of particular interest since they suggest that the illness leaves the patient with an unequivocal deficit as far as normal life is concerned. In a sense, they suggest a circumstance similar to a person who has been in an accident, had an amputation of a leg, and has been ill for a couple of years and finally has learned to live with a certain amount of incapacity. What these case studies do not support is that the individual becomes "well" or "normal" after suffering from chronic schizophrenia. They do, however, suggest improvement in social interaction and capacity to appreciate some life circumstances. It is as if the illness schizophrenia is no longer active but has left an unalterable residue.

In the Iowa 500, 38 of the original schizophrenic patients in the study were rated as having a good psychiatric status at follow-up. This means that, for practical purposes, they were asymptomatic, which meant that the patients showed no symptoms of schizophrenia when they were interviewed using the Iowa Structured Psychiatric Interview (ISPI) (Tsuang et al. 1979). Being asymptomatic does not necessarily mean that the mental status of the proband was normal at the time of the follow-up interview. Of the 382 patients who were given a final diagnosis according to the Feighner criteria, 28 received a final diagnosis of schizophrenia and also were asymptomatic at follow-up around 30–40 years later. Evaluating these patients in light of clinical diagnosis at admission, we found that, of 52 who were clinically diagnosed as paranoid at admission, 16 (31%) were asymptomatic at follow-up 30–40 years later. Of 99 hebephrenics diagnosed clinically at admission, 6 (6%) were asymptomatic. Of 13 diagnosed originally as catatonic, 3 (23%) were asymptomatic, and of 6 who were diagnosed as schizophrenic, uncertain subtype, 3 (50%) were asymptomatic. Thus, having received a clinical diagnosis of hebephrenic schizophrenia made it unlikely, though not impossible, that an individual would end up with no symptoms of schizophrenia in the long-term follow-up. Although only 6% of the hebephrenic patients were asymptomatic at follow-up, 22 of the 71 (31%) schizophrenic patients with other than hebephrenic diagnoses were asymptomatic. Thus, five times as many nonhebephrenic schizophrenic patients had a good psychiatric outcome. These 28 patients are a particularly important group in that they received a Feighner research diagnosis of schizophrenia originally and a follow-up Feighner diagnosis of schizophrenia, thereby fulfilling criteria for schizophrenia according to specific research criteria both at the beginning and at the end of the study. They deserve special attention in order to determine whether their outcome as regards marital status, residential status, and work status was as good as their psychiatric status (defined as a lack of clinical symptoms). Also, the mental status findings, though more subjective and more dependent on the interviewers, can tell us something about their appearance and behavior at the time that they were last seen. It will be important to evaluate them at time of admission and to assess the short-term follow-up material in order to see whether they were more or less likely to have had a remission during that period than those patients who, at the end of long-term follow-up, were still symptomatic.

In order to evaluate the association of outcome variables with the presence of symptoms, we can look at the comparison of the variables of marital status, residential status, and occupational status in the major psychoses (Tsuang et al. 1979). This group evaluates all of the patients for whom follow-up material was available but does not necessarily include only those with a final Feighner diagnosis. There were 38 schizophrenic patients in that group who, it was ascertained, were asymptomatic. In other words, they admitted to no symptoms at all when systematically interviewed. There were 65 schizophrenic patients in that outcome study who enjoyed the best occupational status, which meant that they were either employed or retired or were housewives or students. Assuming that all 38 of the patients also had the best occupational outcome, this leaves 27 (42%) of the patients who had a good work history and who were still symptomatic from their illness. In the case of best residential outcome, which meant that the probands owned their house or lived in a relative's house, we may note that 64 of the schizophrenic patients achieved that level of living. Again, assuming that all 38 of the asymptomatic patients had the best residential record, this leaves 26 (41%) of those with a good residential record as still being ill with the symptoms of schizophrenia. Finally, we have noted that the patients with schizophrenia were less likely to have been married at the time that the study was initiated (at the time of index admission). In the outcome study, 39 had good marital outcome, which meant that they were either married or widowed. This is almost equal to the 38 who were asymptomatic, and it is quite unlikely that all of the schizophrenic patients that were asymptomatic in the follow-up were, in fact, married or widowed. The conclusion that should be drawn is that the living arrangements and the occupational circumstances are not necessarily associated with being psychiatrically well, which is probably also true for the marital status. In the case of good occupational and residential status, no less than 40% of the patients still had to be symptomatic; it is likely that a higher percentage were symptomatic.

In the evaluation of the patients who had a final diagnosis according to the Feighner criteria, there were 170 people who were schizophrenic at follow-up and considered schizophrenic at the time of index admission. Of these, 142 were symptomatic at follow-up by interview, but 28 were asymptomatic. Table 14–1 gives some of the significant differences between the two groups. The group that is asymptomatic after a long-term follow-up was older at time of admission and had a later age at onset. There were fewer patients in the asymptomatic group who had a diagnosis of the hebephrenic subtype of schizophrenia. Symptoms

**Table 14–1.** Comparison of intake variables between followed asymptomatic schizophrenic patients and symptomatic schizophrenic patients

| | Symptomatic at follow-up N = 142 | Asymptomatic at follow-up N = 28 |
|---|---|---|
| Age at admission, ≥ 40 | 3.5 | 21.4 |
| Age first ill, ≥ 30 | 16.2 | 39.3 |
| Previous episodes | 2.8 | 10.7 |
| Initial diagnosis, hebephrenic schizophrenia | 65.5 | 21.4 |
| Initial diagnosis, paranoid schizophrenia | 23.4 | 57.1 |
| Initial diagnosis, other schizophrenia | 9.1 | 21.4 |
| Final diagnosis, hebephrenic schizophrenia | 78 | 43 |
| Final diagnosis, paranoid schizophrenia | 22 | 46 |
| Agitation | 23 | 14 |
| Euphoria | < 1 | 10.7 |
| Pressure of speech | 2.8 | 10.7 |
| Flight of ideas | 0 | 7.1 |
| Nondelusional grandiosity | 2.1 | 14.3 |
| Haptic hallucinations | 27.4 | 48.1 |
| Memory deficit | 14.4 | 3.6 |
| Schizophrenia on maternal and/or paternal side of family | 6 | 0 |
| Hospital diagnosis, paranoid schizophrenia | 21.1 | 39.3 |
| Complete recovery in short-term follow-up | 4.2 | 17.9 |

*Note.*   All values are percentages. All comparisons significantly different at $P = .05$ level or better.

that are seen in mania such as euphoria, pressure of speech, flight of ideas, and nondelusional grandiosity were more frequent in the group that was asymptomatic. Prior episodes were more likely seen in the asymptomatic group, and the asymptomatic group was more likely to have made a recovery in the short-term follow-up period. Thus, the asymptomatic group seems more likely to have an episodic illness than the group that still had symptomatology. Memory deficit was more frequent in the group that continued to be symptomatic, but this group had more haptic hallucinations than the asymptomatic group. The group that was symptomatic at follow-up was more likely to have schizophrenia in an extended family. Agitation was more frequent in the group that was symptomatic, whereas depressive symptoms did not separate the two groups. In general, symptoms that were related to a good psychiatric outcome (i.e., being asymptomatic on a structured interview, which was used to elicit current delusions and hallucinations as well as evidence of thinking problems) were those same kinds of symptoms that were reported years ago. A more episodic illness and the presence of affective, in this case manic, symptoms were associated with a better prognosis, whereas findings such as memory deficit, a schizophrenic family history, and a subtype diagnosis of hebephrenia lent themselves to a poor prognosis. This was true at least for those patients who showed no symptomatology on the interview.

In Table 14–1, we also present the factors that seemed to be related to a good long-term prognosis that was manifested by being asymptomatic. Such factors were euphoria, pressure of speech, flight of ideas, and nondelusional grandiosity. Essentially, these factors describe a picture that is associated with one or more manic symptoms. The second good prognostic item was the presence of previous episodes or complete recovery in a short period of time, which suggested that an episodic course, rather than a chronic downhill course, was associated with being asymptomatic in follow-up. In retrospect, one might give a remitting or a chronic course equal status with the phenomenology of the illness. We then evaluated the frequency of such items in the 142 patients who were considered symptomatic and compared them with the number of good prognosis items that were seen in the 28 patients. For the 142 symptomatic patients, 127 (89%) showed none of these items, whereas 13 of the 28 (46%) showed none of the items. For the symptomatic schizophrenic patients, 13 (9.15%) of the 142 showed one of the items, but one item was shown by 12 of the 28 (43%) of the asymptomatic group. For the presence of two or three symptoms, the symptomatic schizophrenic patients showed this number in .7%, but in the 28 patients, 1 showed two items and 2 showed three items (3.6% and 7%). In a 2 × K chi-square analysis, the difference between the symptomatic versus the nonsymptomatic showing such intake items was significantly different at the .0001 level of probability. A good outcome can be predicted when the patient's diagnosis includes manic affective symptoms or when the patient has had an episodic illness.

One point lacking in prior studies of outcome in schizophrenia is a clear account of the mental status findings at follow-up. In the Iowa 500, a systematic mental status was performed after clinical interview. It consisted of 2 items about the informant's personal appearance, 3 items that describe slowness or reduction of motor activity, 6 items that dealt with agitation or excitement, 11 items that dealt with bizarre behavior, 20 items that dealt with behavioral expression of affect (including expressionless face, inappropriate affect, reduced emotion when delusional or normal material was discussed, failing to answer questions, and verbosity), 1 item about talking to oneself, 14 items concerned with abnormalities of speech, and 10 miscellaneous items that contained observations such as responding without regard to content of questions, disrupting interview, lack of insight, orientation difficulties, and doubtfulness on the part of the interviewer about the credibility of the information in the interview.

Figure 14–1 shows a frequency distribution of the number of mental status findings. Only two patients (7%) had no mental status symptoms at all, and three (11%) had no more than one. Of the 28 patients, 14 had four or fewer mental status findings,

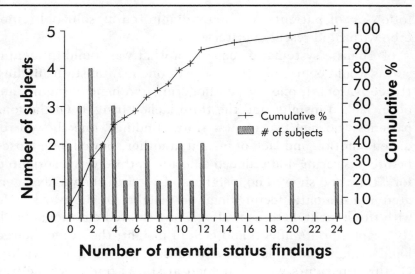

**Figure 14–1.**   Distribution of mental status findings in 28 asymptomatic schizophrenic patients.

whereas the other 14 had five or more. There is an association between having none or one mental status findings at follow-up and having more of the good prognostic signs at index (manic symptoms, episodic course). Four of five (80%) of those with none to one behavioral mental status symptoms had one or more of the good prognostic signs. This was true of 48% (11 of the remaining 23) of those who had two or more mental status findings. Though this is not significant ($P = .074$), the finding suggests that having good prognostic signs such as manic symptoms or an episodic nature of illness is associated with having fewer symptoms at mental status examination 30–40 years later. If one separates the groups at the median (four mental status findings versus five or more) and compares the two groups of 14, 71% of those who had the fewer (four) mental status findings have the good prognostic signs as against five (36%) of those with the many mental status findings ($P = .154$). Though the numbers are small, it appears that an illness with a remitting nature and the symptoms of mania are highly associated with few mental status findings in a 30- to 40-year follow-up of patients originally diagnosed as schizophrenic, even with rigid research criteria.

Perhaps a systematic account of what was found in mental status would be useful. Of those with one mental status finding (three patients), one showed fidgeting and hand wringing, another lacked insight, and the third lacked insight. Of the four patients who had two mental status findings, one showed reduced emotion and lack of insight, another showed long lapses before answering and reduced emotion, a third was disoriented for a time and showed no insight, and a fourth showed exaggerated and dramatic feelings and no insight. Of the two people with three mental status findings, one showed emotional lability, inappropriate affect, and lack of insight; the other showed hand wringing and fidgetiness, verbosity, and circumstantiality. Of three patients with four mental status findings, one was slowed, showed long lapses in response, had no eye contact, and showed abnormal readiness to agree to ideas or commands. Another showed no insight, was verbose, and had a haughty attitude; the interviewer doubted the credibility of the interview. Another showed a lack of insight, verbosity, a loud voice, and reduced emotion. In the remaining 14, there were many more symptoms, including self-neglect, slowness, posturing, no eye contact, reduced emotion, apathy, and failing to answer. Following are the specific symptoms seen in the asymptomatic patients who had five or more mental status findings:

**Patient #4: 12 items.**   Dirty, unkempt, slowed in movements, posturing, avoids looking at interviewer during interview, reduced emotion when delusional or normal material is discussed, emotion not congruent with subject being discussed, apathetic and uninterested, informant fails to answer, sudden and inexplicable interruption of the line of thought without a recognizable reason, informant talks vaguely, preoccupied and inattentive, no insight.

**Patient #5: 15 items.**   Self-neglect, gets up and paces during interview, sings, laughs out of context, unusual and inappropriate behavior, easily distracted, unduly cheerful and smiling, motion not congruent with subject under discussion, joyous mood, talks to self, inappropriate words are associated by the sound of the rhyme, speech incoherent, flight of ideas, interrupts interview, interviewer doubts credibility of information.

**Patient #6:  9 items.**  Self-neglect, unduly cheerful and smiling, abnormal readiness to agree with ideas, apathetic and uninterested, haughty and superior attitude, elated mood, responds without regard to content of questions, interviewer doubts credibility of information, disoriented as to time.

**Patient #7:  7 items.**  Slowed in movements, long lapses before replying, laughs and giggles out of context, blank and expressionless face, reduced emotion when delusional or normal material is discussed, apathetic and uninterested, lacks insight.

**Patient #9:  10 items.**  Posturing, repetitive movements (mannerisms), hallucinatory behavior, perplexity, irritability, apathetic and uninterested, loud voice, talks to self, lacks insight, interviewer doubts credibility of interview.

**Patient #10:  24 items.**  Self-neglect, laughs out of context, unusual and inappropriate behavior, posturing, repetitive movements, facial grimacing, easily distracted, hallucinatory behavior, unduly cheerful and smiling, emotion not congruent with subject under discussion, fails to answer questions, informant talks to self, makes up words that have no accepted meanings, peculiar usage of ordinary words, repetition of interviewer's words (echolalia), incoherent, pedantic manner of speech, frequent repetition of stereotype phrases, speech is tangential and irrelevant, preoccupied and inattentive, responds without regard to content of questions, disoriented as to time, lacks insight, interviewer doubts credibility of interview.

**Patient #13:  20 items.**  Self-neglect, long lapses before replying to questions, mannerisms, hallucinatory behavior, blank and expressionless face, reduced emotion when discussing either delusional or normal material, perplexity, apathetic and uninterested, depressed gloomy mood, monotonous voice, talks to self, makes up words, sudden and inexplicable interruption of a line of thought without obvious reason, incoherent, talks so vaguely that information is of no value, repetition of stereotype phrases, irrelevant speech, preoccupied and inattentive, disoriented in two spheres, lacks insight.

**Patient #14:   10 items.**   Slowed movements, long lapses before replying, lack of movement, easily distracted, reduced emotion in talking about delusional or normal material, low voice hard to hear, failure to answer questions, sudden and inexplicable interruption of a line of thought, lacks insight, interviewer doubts credibility of interview.

**Patient #17:   8 items.**   Unusual and inappropriate behavior, avoids looking at interviewer, hallucinatory behavior, apathetic and uninterested, talks to self, preoccupied and inattentive, disoriented as to place, lacks insight.

**Patient #19:   6 items.**   Long lapses before replying, blank and expressionless face, reduced emotion when discussing delusional or normal material, apathetic and uninterested, informant fails to answer questions, lacks insight.

**Patient #20:   5 items.**   Slow in movement, laughs and giggles out of context, blank and expressionless face, reduced emotion when discussing delusional or normal material, marked changes in speed or volume of voice.

**Patient #23:   12 items.**   The patient paces during interview, laughs and giggles out of context, facial grimacing, is easily distracted, blank and expressionless face, reduced emotion when discussing delusional or normal material, emotion not congruent with subject under discussion, apathetic and uninterested, circumstantial speech, informant continually returns to same subject, no insight, interviewer doubts credibility of interview.

**Patient #24: 7 items.** Blank and expressionless face, reduced emotion when discussing delusional or normal material, apathetic and uninterested, overly suspicious of interviewer, guarded, lacks insight, interviewer doubts credibility of interview.

**Patient #27: 11 items.** Paces during interview, laughs out of context, unusual and inappropriate behavior, facial grimacing, hallucinatory behavior, incoherent speech, informant talks vaguely so that information is of little or no value, tangential and irrelevant, responds without regard to content of questions, lacks insight.

It is important to note that all 14 patients with multiple abnormalities on a mental status examination answered all questions about symptoms in the negative. Though the people who had no symptoms at interview might be considered well, this seems highly unreasonable in view of the fact that they had many symptoms on the mental status evaluation. The reliability studies for the mental status were not as good as the reliability studies for the interview material, but they were shown to be moderately reliable. In grouping behavior ratings, the slowness and retardation mental status findings had an interclass correlation coefficient of .73; bizarre behavior, .76; depressed affect, .71; and a group of items containing the doubt on the part of the interviewer about the credibility of the interview, orientation, and lack of insight, .55. In the case of nine of the patients with no symptoms by interview, the interviewer doubted the credibility of the interview.

Two patients of the 170 final Feighner schizophrenic patients had no symptoms and no mental status findings. This group must be considered well, and it accounts for 1% of the schizophrenic group. Assuming that 14 asymptomatic schizophrenic patients who had four or less mental status findings were well, we would find a total of only 8% are in that class. Data from the Iowa 500 suggest that schizophrenia is a chronic disease that leaves the individual incapacitated either by symptoms that are gained by systematic interview or by mental status findings. This does not mean that the individual cannot work or cannot live independently, but it does suggest that the illness is not one that remits in a total fashion. To this, we might add that the admission clinical symptoms and short-term course findings suggest that some of the patients with a good prognosis may have been misdiagnosed, even though the diagnoses were systematic and reliable in the main.

# Chapter 15

# The Contribution of the Iowa 500 to Diagnosis and Classification of the Affective Disorders and Chronic Nonaffective Psychoses

The criteria that were used to select patients for the Iowa 500 defined syndromes, not necessarily illnesses. These criteria were a beginning but not the final word in defining an illness. It seems that meeting the criteria would be necessary in order to agree that the illness were present but having met the criteria does not in itself make a diagnosis. The symptoms were chosen as criteria because considerable work had already been done indicating that they could be used to predict course and family history in psychiatric patients. Given these criteria as a beginning, it was necessary to select patients; do a systematic family history and systematic family study; assess the follow up in both the long and the short term; and attempt to determine what kinds of outcomes, courses, clinical symptoms, and family history findings cluster together. In a sense, these are the components that make up the definition of the medical model.

The medical model suggests a series of validating factors for the definition of a disease. The first are epidemiologic factors in which certain kinds of illnesses may be particularly related to various demographic variables. As an example, in medicine, Cooley's anemia is seen mainly in a Mediterranean culture and sickle cell anemia in black people. In schizophrenia, there have been data suggesting a downward mobility and an ultimate residence in a low socioeconomic setting because of the illness.

A second factor that can be used in defining a disease is that of premorbid personality. Cyclothymia has often been associated with bipolar illness, and a schizoid personality has been associated with schizophrenia. These are not invariable findings, but they are usually more frequent than one would find in a series of control subjects.

The third factor consists of clinical symptoms and signs of an illness. It would be useful to have a pathognomonic set of symptoms or signs that defined any psychiatric illness. This is found in multiple myeloma, in which the Bence-Jones protein occurs in a certain percentage of the cases. Even though this is unlikely to be helpful in psychiatry, we continue to look for such pathognomonic symptoms and signs. We have yet to find them. In fact, we have very few signs of any kind, but it may be that as we look at some of the material from the Iowa 500 we might find something that approximates pathognomonic symptoms.

The fourth aspect of a disease is course and outcome. This includes both the immediate course; the age at onset; whether or not the patient has an acute, semiacute, or chronic onset; the short-term course of the illness; the short-term outcome; and the long-term course and outcome, which would encompass an individual's entire life. It would also include the stability of the diagnosis and whether or not it might change over time to another, more reasonable, diagnosis.

The fifth aspect of the medical model is that of family history. Patients with diabetes often have diabetes in their family, and patients with Huntington's disease have Huntington's disease in their family; by and large these diseases breed true. Likewise, breeding true is a matter of considerable importance in defining a psychiatric illness. In psychiatric diagnoses, if breeding true were to occur, more depressive subjects would have depression in their family, more manic patients would have mania in their family, and more schizophrenic patients would have schizophrenia in their family. It is important, however, to remember that family history may not be a perfect duplication of the illness of the proband in the family. It may be that certain families with certain kinds of psychiatric illnesses have other psychiatric diagnoses that are found in high frequency when compared to control groups. As an example, a family history of alcoholism may be found to be associated with one or another psychiatric illness.

The sixth factor important for definition of a disease is that of a series of laboratory findings. Although the patients of the Iowa 500 were admitted at a time when laboratory findings and laboratory tests were not common, there were some measurements obtained such as ordinary blood and spinal fluid work. This is, of course, a good part of modern medicine (i.e., the use of laboratory findings), but in psychiatry there is only a beginning in this area. It is necessary to define illnesses using other factors in order to validate the value of the laboratory findings.

Finally, the last aspect in defining a disease is that of response to treatment, which must be specific to be useful. It is entirely possible that some treatment, such as sedation, might be useful in a variety of psychiatric as well as medical circumstances. However, a response to electroconvulsive therapy is clearly more specific to a remitting disease such as mania or depression rather than to a chronic illness such as hysteria, anxiety disorder, or schizophrenia. Lithium also seems to have a specific effect on the treatment and prevention of manic episodes. By use of this medical model and with the access to the data of the Iowa 500, we will attempt to classify the primary affective disorders and some aspects of chronic nonaffective psychoses, specifically those of a nonorganic background.

The data that we have from the Iowa 500 should be relevant to the factors involved in the medical model since there are systematic data on the index syndrome and a clinical diagnosis. Material is available on prior episodes and hospitalization, and, also, data are available on prior personality characteristics. The age at onset and the characteristics of the onset whether acute or chronic are known. The type of onset is generally defined as amount of time from onset to hospitalization. There is a blind family history, which was taken from material that was gleaned by residents, faculty, and social workers, and there was a family study by personal interview that was accomplished 30–40 years after the patient was admitted to the hospital. Most importantly, there is a short-term follow-up, which was essentially untouched by any kind of effective treatment. The depressive and manic patients were admitted to the hospital between 1935 and 1940, prior to the time when electroconvulsive therapy was used at the hospital, and the schizophrenic patients were admitted between 1934 and 1944, prior to the time of any neuroleptic use. The long-term follow-up was done systematically, by personal interview and by amassing a series of clinical materials such as charts from other mental health hospitals. Assessment was made using research criteria about the change in diagnosis or the change in character of the illness. Using the information, it is possible to broadly classify the primary affective disorders and the chronic nonaffective psychoses.

The material of the Iowa 500 allows the classification shown in Figure 15–1. In general, the primary affective disorders tend to be episodic and have remissions and exacerbations, whereas the nonaffective psychoses in this group tend to be chronic and far less variable in their presentation. The affective disorders tend to have major components of mood change such as mania and depression; the chronic nonaffective psychoses tend to have less of this kind of mood change. The schizophrenic patients show incoherent speech, poor social function, motor symptoms, flat or inappropriate affect, and special kinds of delusions and hallucinations, whereas the patients who suffer from the affective disorders have far fewer of these symptoms.

## The Separation of the Primary Affective Disorders From the Chronic Nonaffective Psychoses

Primary affective disorders are manias and/or depressions, which occur independently from an association with a prior psychiatric illness. A secondary affective disorder would be a depression, which occurs after the onset of another nonaffective illness. Such a secondary affective disorder could occur after the patient met criteria for an anxiety disorder, schizophrenia, somatization disorder, organic brain syndrome, or, for that matter, after the onset of a medical disease (Feighner et al. 1972). Considerable research suggests usefulness of separating patients with bipolar disorder (i.e., individuals who have manias and depressions) from the group of affectively ill patients who suffer only from depression (Angst and Perris 1968; Winokur et al. 1969).

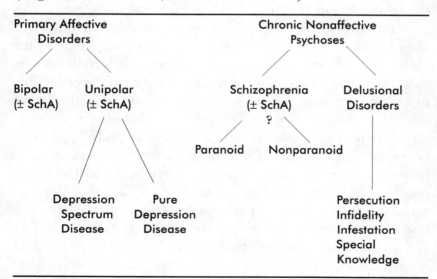

**Figure 15–1.**  Partial disease classification: depression, mania, nonaffective psychoses.

There are clear differences between the primary affective disorders and the chronic nonaffective psychoses as regards symptoms. Table 15–1 gives some of the data that support a separation of the primary affective disorders from the nonaffective psychoses. The clinical symptoms of depression are seen often in unipolar depression and considerably less frequently in the chronic nonaffective psychoses. In fact, in the chronic nonaffective psychoses, the occurrence of depressive symptoms is sporadic, and the patient usually does not meet criteria for a depressive episode except as a secondary condition. A similar occurrence may be seen in separating the bipolar illnesses from the nonaffective psychoses. Again, the symptoms of mania are infrequent in the nonaffective illnesses and, when seen, are sporadic rather than meeting full criteria for an episode. Schizophrenic symptoms, however, are rarely seen in either the unipolar or bipolar affective episodes.

The age at onset of the primary affective disorders is later, as is the age at index admission, compared with the other two samples. Poor premorbid function is more frequently seen in the schizophrenic or chronic nonaffective psychotic group, and prior episodes are more frequently seen in the primary affective disorders. Social incapacity is notable in that the patients with chronic nonaffective psychoses are far more likely to be unmarried. Acuteness of onset is more likely in the primary affective disorders and particularly so in the bipolar patients, but a longer, prodromal, lingering type of onset is more frequent in the chronic nonaffective psychoses. The affectively ill patients are more likely discharged into the community. In a short-term follow-up, complete recovery is rarely seen in the patients with chronic nonaffective psychoses but is seen in about half of the primary affective disorder patients. Deterioration was not seen in the primary affective disorders but is a significant finding in the chronic nonaffective psychoses. The family history of schizophrenia was more likely in the chronic nonaffective psychoses, and the patients with primary affective disorder were more likely to have a history of remitting illness in their family history.

**Table 15–1.** Major differences between patients with unipolar depression, bipolar illness, and chronic nonaffective psychoses

|  | Unipolar<br>N = 98 | Bipolar<br>N = 79 | Chronic<br>nonaffective<br>psychoses<br>N = 167 |
|---|---|---|---|
| Retardation, self-reproach, diurnal variation, anorexia, % | 18–79 | — | .5–17 |
| Euphoria and/or irritability, hyperactivity, pressure of speech, flight of ideas, % | — | 58–70 | 2–6 |
| Passivity delusions, symbolism, blocking and/or mute and/or tangential, flat or inappropriate affect, % | 0–4 | 1–5 | 27–70 |
| Age at onset, median years | 39 | 27 | 24 |
| Age at index admission, median years | 41 | 33 | 28 |
| Poor premorbid function, % | 2 | 6 | 50 |
| Never married, % | 17 | 39 | 72 |
| Antisocial behavior, % | 1 | 3 | 7 |
| One or more prior episodes, % | 43 | 52 | 13 |
| Two or more prior episodes, % | 13 | 16 | 2 |
| Two or more prior admissions, % | 5 | 16 | 8 |
| Length of admission at index admission: |  |  |  |
| 3 months or less, % | 34 | 71 | 3 |
| 3 years or more, % | 4 | 3 | 47 |
| Discharged to community, % | 33 | 37 | 18 |
| One or more subsequent admissions to University of Iowa Psychiatric Hospital, % | 10 | 22 | 9 |
| Complete recovery in short follow-up, % | 45 | 7 | 5 |
| Social recovery or out of hospital, % | 19 | 29 | 13 |
| Never well, socially unrecovered, % | 30 | 14 | 77 |
| Deteriorated, % | 0 | 0 | 13 |

**Table 15–1.** Major differences between patients with unipolar depression, bipolar illness, and chronic nonaffective psychoses *(continued)*

| | Unipolar N = 98 | Bipolar N = 79 | Chronic nonaffective psychoses N = 167 |
|---|---|---|---|
| **Family history in first-degree relatives** | | | |
| Schizophrenia, MR% | .77 | .5 | 1.57 |
| Affective disorder, MR% | 11.5 | 11.9 | 4.7 |
| Extended family history of schizophrenia, % | 3 | 2 | 7 |
| **Long-term follow-up outcome** | | | |
| Single, never married, % | 9 | 22 | 67 |
| Hospitalized in mental hospital, % | 12 | 14 | 18 |
| Own home or with relatives | 70 | 67 | 34 |
| Occupationally incapacitated due to mental illness, % | 17 | 24 | 56 |
| Asymptomatic, % | 61 | 50 | 20 |
| Suicidal, % | 8.7 | 9.7 | 6.4 |
| **Family study** | | | |
| Affective disorder in first-degree relatives, MR% | 12 | 14 | 7 |
| Schizophrenia in first-degree relatives, MR% | 0.9 | 1 | 3 |
| Suicide risk in relatives, % | 3.4 | 1.5 | 1.2 |
| Hospitalized relatives | | | |
| With bipolar illness, % | 20 | 47 | 10 |
| With schizophrenia, % | 12 | 36 | 43 |

*Note.* MR = morbid risk.

The stability of diagnosis over the follow-up period is very striking. If the affective disorders and the chronic nonaffective psychoses did not represent autonomous clinical entities, it would be reasonable for the former to become schizophrenic in follow-up and for some of the chronic nonaffective psychoses to earn the diagnosis of bipolar or unipolar affective disorder over a long period of observation, but diagnostic changes occur infrequently. Of the patients originally diagnosed as schizophrenic, only 4% had a final diagnosis of affective disorder (bipolar or unipolar). Of the affective disorders, only 7% were changed to a diagnosis of schizophrenia in follow-up.

In the long-term follow-up, the patients with chronic nonaffective psychoses were more likely never married and less likely to live in their own home or with relatives, and they were more occupationally incapacitated and less likely to be totally asymptomatic. Like the family history material, the family study material showed that schizophrenia was seen in the primary relatives of the chronic nonaffective psychosis patients and less frequently seen in the families of the primary affective disorder patients. The presence of familial affective disorder was reversed, or more frequently seen in the patients with primary affective disorder.

These data strongly suggest an unequivocal separation of the primary affective disorders from the chronic nonaffective psychoses according to the factors involved in the medical model. Not only are the patients different in terms of clinical picture, which was the point of departure for choosing the groups, but there were also differences in premorbid social characteristics, age at onset, course of illness both in the long- and short-term follow-up, and family history as obtained from both a family history methodology and a family study methodology.

## The Relationship of the Primary Affective Disorders and Chronic Nonaffective Psychoses to the Schizoaffective Syndrome

The schizoaffective syndrome may be either the manic or depressive type. In either case, the patient meets the criteria for a full affective syndrome—be it mania or depression—and during the active phase of the illness has symptoms such as passivity, delusions, thought broadcasting, thought insertion, or withdrawal. These may be called mood incongruent psychotic symptoms, in contrast to mood congruent psychotic symptoms, which would include delusions of sinfulness (seen in depression) or delusions of special abilities (seen in mania).

An early attempt to assess the place of schizoaffective disorder in the scheme of things was accomplished by Tsuang and Dempsey (1979). Of the 315 patients who received a clinical diagnosis of schizophrenia but who did not meet Feighner criteria for schizophrenia, Tsuang and Dempsey took 85 who had both schizophrenic and affective features at time of admission. These patients were compared with the schizophrenic, the manic, and the depressive patients who met Feighner criteria in the Iowa 500 for the purpose of determining the diagnostic placement of schizoaffective disorder. For a combined outcome, the schizoaffective subjects were significantly different from the those who were schizophrenic, manic, and depressive. More specifically, however, there were comparisons for marital, residential, and occupational status. For marital and residential status, the schizophrenic patients of the Iowa 500 were significantly worse than those who were schizoaffective, but the schizoaffective subjects were equal to those who were manic and depressive. Regarding occupational status, the schizoaffective subjects were the same as those who were schizophrenic and manic but significantly worse than those who were depressive. For psychiatric status, there was no difference between the subjects who were schizoaffective and schizophrenic, but, after 30–40 years, schizoaffective patients were significantly worse than either the manic or the depressive patients. The authors concluded that the schizoaffective disorder patients fell somewhere in between the schizophrenia and the mania group.

Coryell and Tsuang (1979) evaluated the family histories of the schizophrenic, manic, and depressive probands in the Iowa 500 and compared those family histories with 310 of 315 schizophrenic patients who were clinically diagnosed but did not meet the Feighner criteria for schizophrenia. These "non-Feighner" schizophrenic subjects contained the group of 85 who had been diagnosed as having schizoaffective disorder. The 310 non-

Feighner schizophrenic probands had a morbid risk for schizophrenia in first-degree relatives of 2.25%, and this was significantly higher than the morbid risk for schizophrenia in the depressive probands (.41%). However, the non-Feighner schizophrenic probands were not significantly different from the schizophrenic probands or the manic probands regarding a family history of schizophrenia. For affective disorder, the schizophrenic probands had a significantly lower morbid risk (5.5%) than the non-Feighner schizophrenic probands (8.6%). Likewise, the depressive probands had a higher family history of affective disorder in their first-degree relatives (14.32%) than the non-Feighner schizophrenic patients. However, the manic probands did not significantly differ from the non-Feighner schizophrenic probands. How many of these patients might be considered schizoaffective depends on a definition of schizoaffective disorder. Certainly some would fit the criteria of schizoaffective disorder as noted previously. The cutting point here is that schizophrenic patients who did not meet the Feighner criteria are not typical of those diagnosed with schizophrenia, and they are somehow in between the affective disorder and schizophrenia as regards family history.

For the 85 patients who were considered schizoaffective in the long-term follow-up study described previously, Tsuang and associates (1976) looked at them specifically. They had chosen these patients because they had many affective symptoms or they had a remitting course, though they had received a clinical diagnosis of schizophrenia. There were more females among the schizoaffective disorder patients than among the schizophrenic patients, which makes them more similar to the sex ratios in the affective disorders. This was significant, but so was the fact that there was a significant increase in females when compared with the unipolar patients, whereas the male-to-female ratio between bipolar and schizoaffective patients was not significantly different. Regarding short-term recovery, 58% of bipolar and unipolar patients showed this, and only 8% of schizophrenic patients. Schizoaffective patients showed recovery in 44%, making them considerably more similar to the affective disorder patients than to the schizophrenic patients. The family history of schizophrenia was significantly lower in the unipolar group compared with schizoaffective patients (.4% versus 1.3%). However, the same amount of schizophrenia in the families of the schizoaffective patients was found in the family members of the schizophrenic patients (1.3%). Regarding the family history of affective disorder in the schizoaffective patients, occurrence was significantly greater than for the schizophrenic patients, and the family history of affective disorder in the schizoaffective subjects was very similar to that of the primary affective disorder patients (bipolar plus unipolar). These findings suggest that, in this group of 85 schizoaffective patients, there was a closer relationship to affective disorder than to schizophrenia.

Relevant to the question of the appropriate place and classification of schizoaffective disorder is the role of psychotic features in major depression. Coryell and associates (1982) evaluated the importance of mood congruence in psychotic features in major depression. As a preliminary, these authors reevaluated the early family history data of the Iowa 500 in order to determine how reliable obtaining a family history might be by two different observers. The agreement was great for both schizophrenia and for affective disorder.

Of 225 unipolars, 122 had delusions and/or hallucinations, and, of these, 16.4% had mood congruent psychotic features according to DSM-III definitions. The study also included the 310 non-Feighner schizophrenic subjects who met DSM-III criteria for major unipolar depression. Of the pooled groups, the morbid risks for familial affective disorder were as follows: for nonpsychotic major depression, 13%; for mood congruent psychotic major depression, 13%; for mood incongruent major depression, 8%; for schizophreniform disorders, 7%; and for schizophrenia, 6%. In affective disorder, there was a significant lowering of familial affective disorder in the mood incongruent major depressive patients as compared with the nonpsychotic major depressive patients. The authors concluded that morbid risks for familial affective disorder and schizophrenia distinguished mood incongruent patients from nonpsychotic depressive but not from schizophrenic patients. The mood congruent major depressive subjects were more like nonpsychotic depressive subjects. These data, then, unlike the material from Tsuang and co-workers (1976), did not as clearly differentiate the schizoaffective from the schizophrenic subjects. The mood congruent major depressive patients would have many similarities to the schizoaffective patients in the Tsuang and co-workers (1976) study. Coryell and Tsuang (1982) evaluated the importance of delusions in primary unipolar depression. In the short-term follow-up, the nondelusional patients were more likely to recover than were the delusional primary unipolar depressive patients. A large percentage of them, in fact, had mood incongruent symptomatology; however, not all did. In the 40-year follow-up, the delusional depressive patients showed no difference in marital, occupational, residential, or psychiatric status from the nondelusional depressive patients, but both were different from the schizophrenic patients. The comparisons leave something to be desired as regards a decision on the nature of schizoaffective disorder.

The Iowa 500 data does not provide a clean answer as to whether or not schizoaffective disorder is mainly related to affective disorder or to schizophrenia or to whether it is a third, independent psychosis. Newer data summarized by Winokur (1991) suggest that there are two types of schizoaffective disorder: one is a secondary depression to an ongoing process of schizophrenia and the second, a unipolar/bipolar affective disorder that manifests itself by mood incongruent symptomatology mixed with the affective symptomatology. The two groups are separated by the primary schizophrenic patients having a subacute or chronic course and a lack of episodes. The affective type of schizoaffective disorder manifests itself by having a very acute course over a few months and a follow-up course of episodes. Interestingly, this way of looking at schizoaffective disorder depends less on the clinical symptoms and more on the course of the illness. The study of schizoaffective disorder is very important because, ultimately, it will define the boundary between schizophrenia and affective disorder.

## The Partial Classification of
## the Affective Disorders

The starting point for the classification of the affective disorders is the separation of bipolar from unipolar illness. Bipolar illness is defined as an affective disorder in which mania occurs. There may or may not be depressions associated with the manias, but usually these do appear. Unipolar illness manifests itself by simple unipolar depressions. From Table 15–1, it is clear that bipolar patients have an earlier age at onset and an earlier age at admission, and they have a more episodic illness in that they have more subsequent admissions. The onset of their illness is more rapid than the onset in the unipolar depressive patients, and this is very striking. Of course, there are differences in symptoms in that the bipolar patients have more manic symptoms and the unipolar patients lack these. On the other hand, relatively few differences exist between the depressions that are seen in bipolar illness and those seen in unipolar illness.

Patients who are admitted with a unipolar depression become bipolar; that is, they show mania in about 10% of the cases (Winokur and Wesner 1987). Patients who develop a mania over a period of time differ from the patients who are stable unipolar in that the former have a history of more episodes prior to their onset of mania, more hospital admissions, more marked self-reproach, and more guilt. Most studies show that more relatives of bipolar probands have an affective illness when compared with the relatives of unipolar probands, though the difference in risks in the Iowa 500 was not significantly different. In deceased first-degree relatives of bipolar patients versus relatives of unipolar depressed patients, more relatives had a hospitalization for bipolar illness (40%) than was seen in the unipolar relatives (20%). These findings are consistent with prior findings in the separation of bipolar from unipolar illness in that the bipolar patients have more bipolar family members than are found in unipolar patients. Altogether, the contribution of the Iowa 500 supports differences between bipolar patients in onset and course as well as in a family history of mania.

The separation of the large mass of unipolar depressions into endogenous and reactive or neurotic has had a long and disputatious history. In an effort to classify unipolar depression into meaningful subtypes, Winokur and associates (1971) evaluated two large groups of the primary unipolar depressive patients. This study showed that early onset patients were more likely to have alcoholism and antisocial personality in their first-degree relatives than were late onset depressive patients. Early onset depressive patients (those with an illness beginning before age 40) showed an increased propensity for first-degree female family members to be depressed than first-degree male family members. Also, there was a larger amount of affective disorder and depression in the families of early onset depressive patients. In general, the early onset depressive patients have more psychopathology (all kinds) in first-degree family members than did the older onset group. Ultimately, a familial subtyping was attempted, which dealt with two groups: depression spectrum disease, which is an ordinary depression in a person who had a family history of alcoholism and pure depressive disease, which is a depression in a person in whom there was no evidence of alcoholism or antisocial personality in the family (Winokur et al. 1982). To this separation of the familial subtypes—depression spectrum disease and pure depressive disease—the Iowa 500 study made a considerable contribution. Specifically, the variables that separated depression spectrum patients from pure depressive disease patients were that the former had an earlier onset, were younger at admission, and were more likely female (because the males in the family had a primary alcoholism).

Other related findings concern gender differences. There were significant increases in agitation and precipitating factors in females and a significant increase in retardation in males. Patients with early onset of unipolar depression were more likely to be discharged to the community, were more likely retarded, and were more likely to suffer from diurnal variation, whereas late onset patients were more likely to be agitated. For young patients (younger than 40 years), retardation was more frequent, and young patients differed from older patients in that they were less likely agitated and less likely ill for a period of 6 months or more at index admission (Winokur et al. 1973).

Finally, using material from five series of unipolar depressed patients, one series of which was the Iowa 500 unipolar group, Cadoret and co-workers (1977) investigated the relationship of age at onset in unipolar affective disorder to the risk of alcoholism. A break-point model was used, and the risks for alcoholism in relatives of female unipolar probands showed a sharp drop for female probands with an onset age of greater than 40. The alcoholism risk findings were compatible with a two-disease hypothesis, one type of which would be a unipolar depression associated with familial alcoholism.

Table 15–2 presents data on a separation of primary unipolar depressive patients based on the presence and absence of a family history of alcoholism. Of course the presence of a family history of alcoholism defines depression spectrum disease and the absence defines pure depressive disease. Depression spectrum disease is an ordinary primary depression for which the use of the word "spectrum" is relevant to the fact that such families have a spectrum of psychiatric illnesses, which include both depression and alcoholism and antisocial personality in some studies. From the table, one may note that females are more likely to have alcoholic fathers, and this is particularly true of early onset females (i.e., women who had the onset of their depression before age 40). Chronicity of the depression is uncommon if a depressed patient has an alcoholic father. The onset of the illness is more likely acute in patients who lack alcoholism in their first-degree family members. In fact, an abrupt onset, an onset that is 1 month prior to the hospitalization, is four times as frequent in patients who have no family history of alcoholism. Thus, pure depressive disease is much more likely related to an acute onset. These kinds of data were very useful separating depression spectrum disease from familial pure depressive disease. Subsequent studies have shown that the depression spectrum patients have many more problems with normal living and personal difficulties than do pure depressive disease patients (Winokur 1991). Such data as have been gathered from studies like the Iowa 500 suggest that depression spectrum disease is a primary depression usually, but not invariably, in a woman with a long history of stormy life problems and personality difficulties. A family history of alcoholism then usefully describes a particular kind of depressed patient. These findings are meaningful in terms of potential treatment strategies.

It is possible to divide the pure depressive disease patients into two groups, one in which there is a family history of depression and another in which the family history is completely nega-

**Table 15–2.** Relationship of a family history of alcoholism to some characteristics of depressive patients

|  | Morbid risk for alcoholism in fathers |
| --- | --- |
| Females | 15.4 |
| Males | 5.2 |
| Early age at onset, females ≤ 40 | 19 |
| Late age at onset, males > 40 | 5 |
|  | Fathers alcoholic |
| Chronic unipolar depressive patients | 2 |
| Nonchronic unipolar depressive patients | 15 |
|  | Duration of illness ≤ 3 months prior to hospitalization |
| Depression spectrum patients | 22 |
| Pure depressive disease patients | 39 |
|  | Abrupt onset 1 month prior to hospitalization |
| Depression spectrum patients | 3 |
| Pure depressive disease patients | 13 |

*Note.* All values are percentages.

tive, which would leave us with two new groups: one called familial pure depressive disease (FPDD) and the other called sporadic depressive disease (SDD). The simple fact that an individual does not have a family history of affective disorder does not mean that the illness is not genetic. It means that the illness has not manifested itself in a family member for what may be a variety of reasons. By use of data from the Iowa 500, a comparison was made between 48 female patients with FPDD and 45 patients who had similar depressions but had a negative family history, qualifying them for the diagnosis of SDD. The index age in both groups was the same, 45–46 years, but the age at onset in the patients with SDD was significantly older, 42 versus 35. Also, a large number of the patients with SDD had an insidious onset that lasted for a period of 2 years before they were hospitalized (22%). Marked guilt was more frequently seen in the patients with FPDD than in the patients with SDD ($P = .025$). There were no other obvious symptom differences; however, patients with SDD did stay in the hospital for longer than 3 months more frequently than did the patients with FPDD, suggesting that SDD is a more lingering illness both in onset as well as in period of hospitalization. In follow-up, there were no differences in terms of numbers of subsequent episodes, chronicity, or hospitalizations. Both groups showed complete recovery in the same number of patients (44%–46%). Thus, there are some differences in FPDD versus SDD when controlled for age and sex; however, they are not striking, and there is no strong or compelling reason to consider them as separate diseases.

## The Classification of the Chronic Nonaffective Psychoses

The classification of the chronic nonaffective psychoses poses particular problems, and there are two aspects of it that deserve mention. First, as implied, these psychoses are chronic, possibly never completely remitting. Such patients may have exacerbations and may improve in behavior and symptoms, but these changes occur in the context of demonstrable mental status aberrations. Exacerbations may be related to adverse circumstances. Once the illness begins, the course may be downhill or stable, or there may be some improvement over years, but from the data presented in Chapter 13 it is unlikely that the patient will achieve total wellness or will be totally free from the symptoms of the illness. Second, they are nonaffective in that the number of affective symptoms is minimal and, if present, may be considered as a secondary phenomenon that occurs in the context of the basic illness. The chronic nonaffective psychoses may show a secondary depressive syndrome at certain points during the chronic illness. On occasion, some chronically ill patients show some symptoms of mania, usually garrulousness, but rarely a full manic syndrome. Often, there is a dissociation of the affect and the other manic symptoms, with the affect appearing flat in the presence of overtalkativeness and overactivity. Likewise, in the chronic nonaffective psychoses, mood incongruent psychotic symptoms appear in the absence of a depressive syndrome or manic symptoms. There are some patients with affective disorder, either bipolar or unipolar, who have periods of chronicity. These periods may last a long time, but there is a strong tendency for them to remit over years.

Like the affective illnesses, the chronic nonaffective psychoses are sometimes associated with organic cerebral disorders (Davison 1983), which has been noted for the following reason: schizophrenia occurs in the course of many organic cerebral disorders with a greater than chance expectancy. Though there may be some symptom differences, these schizophrenia-like psychoses associated with organic cerebral disorders generally express symptoms that are not dissimilar to spontaneously occurring psychoses that are diagnosed as schizophrenia. The organic chronic nonaffective psychosis is not associated with a genetic loading for schizophrenia. The site of the brain lesion may be important in the patients who show these psychoses, as noted by Davison, who particularly mentions lesions in the temporal lobe and diencephalon. Similarly, there are affective psychoses associated with organic cerebral disorders where presumably different loci in the brain will turn out to be involved. Schizophrenia (chronic nonaffective psychoses) and affective illnesses differ in another fashion. Though there are good data suggesting a "reactive depression" to occurrences such as death of a close relative or friend, serious medical disorder not affecting the brain, natural tragedies, and hard economic times, there are few data to support a "reactive schizophrenia" or a reactive chronic nonaffective psychosis.

The Iowa 500 did not deal with the organic schizophrenia and other organic chronic nonaffective psychoses. Davison, reviewing Huntington's disease, showed an increased prevalence of both the schizophrenic-type psychoses as well as an increased prevalence of paranoid psychoses (essentially paranoid hallucinatory psychoses resembling paranoid schizophrenia) in patients with Huntington's disease. However, the Iowa 500 primarily dealt with patients who had idiopathic types of chronic nonaffective psychoses. It is possible to present a preliminary classification of the nonorganic types of chronic nonaffective psychoses from the data in the Iowa 500; however, at this point, more work needs to be done.

Partial classification of the chronic nonaffective psychoses contains four entities: 1) delusional disorder, 2) hallucinatory delusional disorder, 3) paranoid schizophrenia, and 4) hebephrenic-catatonic or nonparanoid schizophrenia. The two conditions on the outside of the classification, simple delusional disorder and hebephrenic-catatonic schizophrenia, are clearly different from each other. Some argument may support the possibility that hallucinatory delusional disorder bears a relationship with simple delusional disorder, and paranoid schizophrenia is simply a milder form of a generic schizophrenia, which would include, as the more severe form, the hebephrenic-catatonic type. Table 15–3 presents characteristics of the four groups.

Prior to defining the four groups, several points are important concerning the study of the Iowa 500. First, the Feighner

**Table 15–3.** Classification of chronic nonaffective psychoses including simple and hallucinatory delusional disorder and paranoid and hebephrenic-catatonic schizophrenia

| Defining characteristics | SDD | HDD | PS | HCS |
|---|---|---|---|---|
| Chronic | + | + | + | + |
| Delusions, implausible | + | + | + | + |
| Hallucinations | – | + | + | + |
| Delusions, impossible | – | – | + | + |
| Thought disorder | – | – | – | + |
| Flat affect (masklike) | – | – | – | + |
| Inappropriate affect | – | – | – | + |
| Motor symptoms | – | – | – | + |
| Avolition | – | – | – | + |

Synonyms
SDD/paranoia

HDD/NE, paranoia, affect-laden paraphrenia, paraphrenia, paranoid state, involutional paranoid state

HCS/chronic nonparanoid schizophrenia

| Validators | SDD | HDD | PS | HCS |
|---|---|---|---|---|
| Premorbidly jealous, persecutory | + | + | No | NE |
| Family history of paranoid syndromes, secrecy, jealousy, suspiciousness | 27% | NE | 0% | NE |
| Paranoid disorder in relatives | + | – | – | NE |
| Relatives secretive, jealous, suspicious | + | NE | – | – |
| Schizophrenia symptoms in follow-up | – | NE | + | + |
| No new diagnosis | + | NE | + | + |
| Discharged to community | + | NE | – | – |
| Age at admission | 41 | NE | 27–34 | 27–34 |
| Paranoid, premorbid | 10% | 11% | 4% | NE |
| Jealous, premorbid | 7% | 0% | 1% | NE |
| Schizoid, premorbid | 1% | 3% | 5% | NE |
| Erotic delusions | 3% | 11% | 12% | NE |
| Persecutory delusions | + | + | 100% | 84% |
| Somatic delusions | 2% | 5% | 20% | NE |
| Systematized delusions | 81% | 47% | 32% | NE |
| Jealous delusions | 43% | 21% | 11% | NE |

**Table 15–3.** Classification of chronic nonaffective psychoses including simple and hallucinatory delusional disorder and paranoid and hebephrenic-catatonic schizophrenia (*continued*)

| Validators | SDD | HDD | PS | HCS |
|---|---|---|---|---|
| Grandiose delusions | 2% | 18% | 9% | 12% |
| Hypochondriacal delusions | 7% | 5% | 14% | NE |
| Religious delusions | 3% | 8% | 14% | |
| Familial schizophrenia | – | NE | + | + |
| Short-term outcome, improved from records | NE | NE | 29% | 11% |
| Occupational outcome, better | NE | NE | 64% | 28% |
| Residential outcome, better | NE | NE | 61% | 23% |
| Psychiatric outcome, better | NE | NE | 64% | 38% |

*Note.* SDD = simple delusional disorder; HDD = hallucinatory delusional disorder; PS = paranoid schizophrenia; HCS = hebephrenic-catatonic schizophrenia; NE = not evaluated; – = negative; + = positive.

criteria do not separate delusional disorder from schizophrenia (Feighner et al. 1972). The diagnosis of schizophrenia requires a chronic illness of at least 6 months of symptoms prior to the index evaluation, without return to a premorbid level of psychosocial adjustment, and the absence of a period of depressive or manic symptoms sufficient to qualify for affective disorder or probable affective disorder. This second point has been variously dealt with by different investigators. Some investigators using the Iowa 500 find that a clearly secondary depression does not obviate the diagnosis of schizophrenia, while others accept the simple statement that there must be a clear absence of enough criteria to qualify for either a manic or depressive diagnosis. The other criteria for schizophrenia include delusions or hallucinations without significant perplexity or disorientation associated with them where such delusions or hallucinations could be quite systematized. If there were only systematized delusions, all of which were of an implausible but not impossible type, the patient could, in fact, qualify for a diagnosis of delusional disorder or paranoia. There are, of course, other symptoms such as incoherent language or difficult-to-understand communications. Such symptoms would clearly take patients either out of delusional disorder or the paranoid schizophrenia type and put them into the hebephrenic-catatonic type (Tsuang and Winokur 1974). In a sense, then, the diagnoses are made by exclusion from right to left in Table 15–3. As noted in the table, delusional disorder has the least number of symptoms. Other items that would be in favor of schizophrenia would be a single marital status, poor premorbid social adjustment or work history, a family history of schizophrenia in the absence of alcoholism or drug abuse, and an onset of the illness prior to the age of 40. None of these items could be used to separate schizophrenia from delusional disorder. Thus, there is a good possibility that some of the patients in the Iowa 500 had delusional disorder, and, in fact, an evaluation of the group of schizophrenic patients shows that this is so.

Winokur (1977) presented some criteria for delusional disorder (paranoia) that included exhibiting an unequivocal delusion. Such a delusion or delusions could have been present for any length of time, and the delusion had to be related to events that were possible, although implausible. Thus, a delusion about infidelity or being persecuted by a law agency was possible, but a delusion about being from another planet was unacceptable. The presence or suggestion of any hallucination at any time, bizarre or fantastic; evidence of organic brain syndrome; illness beginning after age 60; meeting clear criteria for depression or mania; and inappropriateness or marked flattening of affect were exclusion criteria in delusional disorder.

In a study of delusional disorder of the simple type, Winokur (1977) evaluated 29 patients who met the above criteria. The findings included patients having a normal intelligence quotient. Seventy-three percent of the patients had an onset between ages 30 and 50 years, considerably older than the onset in patients with hebephrenic-catatonic schizophrenia. The length of illness at onset or at index admission was greater than 1 year in 74% of the delusional disorder patients. The major themes that were seen in the patients with delusional disorder were conjugal problems (conjugal paranoia), legal problems, litigious problems, sexual problems, being unfairly treated or plotted against, and special scientific ability. Of the 29 patients, 11 had conjugal paranoia, and 10 had delusional disorder related to being unfairly treated or plotted against. The other kinds of problems were relatively uncommon as shown by patients with satisfactory work history (75%). It was difficult to determine real precipitating factors, and, personality-wise, 45% were considered embittered, 21% haughty, 17% fussy or rigid, and 66% jealous or suspicious. Regarding nondelusional symptoms, there were very few depressive symptoms, and these patients did not meet the criteria for an affective illness. They showed a high frequency of sexual problems, and they often showed at least one manic symptom that generally was overtalkativeness or circumstantiality (30% of all cases). Most patients were discharged to the community in contrast to the schizophrenic patients, for whom the course was a transfer to another hospital. Specifically, the major symptoms seen in these patients were delusions of reference (76%), delusions of jealousy (48%), delusions of persecution (83%), delusions of a hypochondriacal nature (10%), and delusions of grandeur with great ability in science (7%). Again, note that 48% showed at least one manic symptom, and, in follow-up, 69% were considered chronically ill. The follow-up was a relatively short period of time, but some were followed for a long period. About 31% were considered socially recovered, but whether or not these patients were asymptomatic is unknown. In 93%, there was no new diagnosis, but in 3% a diagnosis of schizophrenia was given; in 3%, affective disorder was a final diagnosis. Sixty-one percent did productive work since discharge, and half of the patients had a stable marriage. Schizophrenic symptoms in the follow-up were not seen in 96%. We have gone into some depth describing these patients in that it is important that they be separated from the group of schizophrenic patients.

There is a lot of evidence that schizophrenia and delusional disorder are separate and autonomous groups. Kendler and co-workers (1981) showed that probands with DSM-III–type schizophrenia do not have an increased incidence of delusional disorder in their relatives. Winokur (1985) showed that patients with delusional disorder did not have an increased incidence of schizophrenic relatives. These findings considered together suggest that schizophrenia and delusional disorder (paranoia) breed true and should be separated from one another.

The relevance of the Iowa 500 to the discussion of delusional disorder and schizophrenia is clear. Several estimates of the study group have shown that there is some contamination in the schizophrenia with paranoia. Kendler noted (personal communication) that, according to DSM-III criteria, none of the Iowa 500 patients could be diagnosed as having delusional disorder, but he did code another classification, which was delusional disorder that did not meet DSM-III criteria. He separated them into simple delusional disorder (that group with delusions but no hallucinations) and hallucinatory delusional disorder (that group with implausible but not impossible delusions and hallucinations). He found that there were five patients with simple delusional disorder and two patients with hallucinatory delusional disorder. Winokur (1985) evaluated 29 patients of the Iowa 500 who had a diagnosis of paranoid schizophrenia according to the Feighner criteria at index and also had a diagnosis of paranoid schizophrenia at follow-up. These were specifically studied, and at index 10 of them met the criteria for delusional disorder according to what has been described previously (Winokur 1977). Finally, Crowe and co-workers (1988) investigated the subject of delusional disorder, and many of the cases he studied overlapped with the Iowa 500 cases. So, the schizophrenic patients of the Iowa 500 contributed a great deal to this particular classification, though, in fact, those patients were not the only patients who made up the classification.

The differentiation between simple delusional disorder and hebephrenic-catatonic schizophrenia, both of which are chronic nonaffective psychoses, is nevertheless distinct. There are differences in definition since simple delusional disorder has implausible delusions but not impossible delusions and hebephrenic-catatonic schizophrenia has both. Such negative symptoms as flat affect, inappropriate affect, and avolition are seen in hebephrenic-catatonic schizophrenia, but they are not seen in simple delusional disorder. The synonym for simple delusional disorder is paranoia, which has never been used to describe hebephrenic-catatonic schizophrenia. In addition to the definitional differences, there are differences in family history. Hebephrenic-catatonic schizophrenia includes a family history of schizophrenia, and simple delusional disorder includes a family history of paranoid psychoses and traits such as secrecy, jealousy, and suspiciousness in family members (Kendler et al. 1985a; Winokur 1985, 1985a). In fact, there may be some reason to postulate a delusional disorder spectrum that would cover both simple delusional disorder as well as paranoid personality traits such as the ones described above. This spectrum has been presented by Rogers and Winokur (1988). The schizophrenia spectrum would be different from the delusional disorder spectrum and would contain schizotypal personality disorder, schizophrenia, and probably schizoid personality. In addition, various kinds of personality problems and minor psychiatric illnesses may also be seen in schizophrenia (Winokur et al. 1972).

The only study that deals with a differentiation on a clinical level among simple delusional disorder, hallucinatory delusional disorder, and paranoid schizophrenia has been done by Crowe. This is unpublished, but, with Dr. Crowe's permission, we are presenting some of the data in this book (Table 15–3). Crowe studied 101 patients with simple delusional disorder, 38 hallucinatory delusional disorder patients, and 118 paranoid schizophrenic patients, which included a considerable overlap with the patients of the Iowa 500. The patients with simple delusional disorder were unmarried only in 19% of the cases, but the patients with hallucinatory delusional disorder and paranoid schizophrenic patients were single in 32% and 43% of the cases, respectively. The patients with simple delusional disorder were more likely employed at time of index than either of the other two groups, but the hallucinatory delusional disorder patients were more like the simple delusional disorder patients than the paranoid schizophrenic patients. There were also personality differences where persecutory premorbid personality traits were seen both in the patients with simple delusional disorder and hallucinatory delusional disorder as opposed to the paranoid schizophrenic patients. Jealousy, however, was only seen essentially in the patients with simple delusional disorder, and schizoid personality was more frequent in the paranoid schizophrenics. Persecutory delusions were more frequent in patients with hallucinatory delusional disorder and the paranoid schizophrenia group, but jealousy delusions were twice as frequent in the simple delusional disorder group as the hallucinatory delusional disorder group and four times as frequent than in the paranoid schizophrenic group. Grandiosity was most frequent in the hallucinatory delusional disorder group. Erotic delusions were seen in only 3% of the simple delusional group, but in 11% of the hallucinatory delusional disorder group and 12% of the paranoid schizophrenic group. Religious delusions were seen in 3% of the simple delusional disorder group, 8% of the hallucinatory delusional disorder group, and 14% of the paranoid schizophrenic group. Somatic delusions were seen only in 2% of the simple delusional disorder group, 5% of the hallucinatory delusional disorder group, and 20% of the paranoid schizophrenic group. All of the hallucinatory delusional disorder group had hallucinations, but only 75% of the paranoid schizophrenic group did, which, of course, would have excluded patients from the simple delusional disorder group. Regarding outcome, 80% of the simple delusional disorder group were home compared with 68% of the hallucinatory delusional disorder group and 59% of the paranoid schizophrenic group. Twenty-seven percent of the simple delusional disorder group, 16% of the hallucinatory delusional disorder group, and 14% of the paranoid schizophrenic group were considered "recovered." In a blind family history, paranoid disorder was seen in 2.3% of the simple delusional disorder group, but only in 1.1% of the hallucinatory delusional disorder group and .6% of the paranoid schizophrenic group. There were no differences in affective disorder. Schizophrenia was seen in .5% of the simple delusional disorder group, 1.8% of the hallucinatory delusional disorder group, and 1.5% of the paranoid schizophrenic group. Paranoid personality in relatives was more frequently seen in the simple delusional disorder group than in the other two groups, but the hallucinatory delusional disorder group was in between. Crowe et al. (1988) also compared jealous and nonjealous types of delusional disorder. The jealous patients experienced a more benign course as indicated by a lower rate of hospitalization and outpatient treatment. The nonjealous patients were mainly patients with delusional disorder of the paranoid type. All of the patients had only simple delusional disorder. At follow-up, of 37 jealous patients, 17 had jealous delusions, but none of the 51 nonjealous patients had jealous delusions. The family history suggested the paranoid disorders were seen equally in both of the two groups. There was no difference in either schizophrenia or affective disorder. Schizophrenia was seen in .3% of the first-degree family members of the jealous group and in .6% family members of the nonjealous group. This amount of familial schizophrenia is similar to the amount expected in the general population.

Though the content of delusional disorder is mainly persecution or infidelity, there are other types. In addition to delusions of high descent and delusions of having special knowledge, some patients manifest delusions of infestation or parasitosis. These patients believe, with an alterable conviction, that there are organisms under their skin. If such syndromes include tactile hallucinations, they would have to be considered as hallucinatory delusional disorder. But, if hallucinations are absent, the diagnosis would be that of simple delusional disorder. Delusional infestation may be another large group that deserves to be considered separately. These symptoms are generally not seen by psychiatrists but rather by dermatologists. Whether the family background includes paranoid syndromes, suspiciousness, jealousy, or secrecy has yet to be studied in any depth. A preliminary report by Kushon and co-workers (1991) estimates 7,100–19,800 new cases of delusional parasitism each year in the United States; females predominate, with a female-to-male ratio of 2.6:1, and most patients are employed. Abnormal paranoid personality traits were identified in this study of 93 patients. Suffice it to say that there may be several different types of delusional disorder that do not necessarily have to be related to each other.

We may conclude from the data that simple delusional disorder is clearly different from either paranoid schizophrenia and hebephrenic-catatonic schizophrenia; however, the hallucinatory delusional disorder patients seemed to be in between, and they may include some patients that belong in either one of the two flanking groups, simple delusional disorder or paranoid schizophrenia.

The separation of paranoid schizophrenia from hebephrenic-catatonic schizophrenia is another problem entirely. Kendler and co-workers (1984) compared the outcome of the schizophrenia subtypes and found that there was clear evidence that paranoid schizophrenia had a better outcome both in the short term as well as the long term. However, in a family study of subtypes of schizophrenia from the Iowa 500, Kendler and colleagues (1988) showed no significant differences existed. Certainly, paranoid schizophrenic patients have an older age at onset and a more benign course, but, for us to consider them as having a separate illness, it would be necessary to find a clear familial difference. This has not been found in the Iowa 500, though other studies have suggested this, and we are left with the possibility that hebephrenic-catatonic schizophrenia is simply a more severe form of schizophrenia with no known reason to say this. The data, however, clearly show a difference between simple delusional disorder and hebephrenic-catatonic schizophrenia and also between simple delusional disorder and paranoid schizophrenia. Thus, there may be two or, possibly, four subtypes of chronic nonaffective psychoses. Considering the clinical syndrome, the course of illness, and the family history, it is feasible to suspect that there are more than two types of illness in the chronic nonaffective psychoses, but only further research will clarify the problem and provide a final answer. The classification described in this chapter differs from other systems that have propounded (e.g., Feighner criteria, DSM-III and

DSM-III-R criteria, RDC). Though this classification is partial, it does have the advantage of being data-bound and conforming to a medical model of disease.

In summary, regarding classification and knowledge of psychiatric illnesses, we have made considerable progress, and the Iowa 500 has contributed to this. It has presented new ways of investigating clinical entities and familial illness, and it has employed systematic and rigorous diagnostic criteria, but, most importantly, it has dealt with patients who were virtually untreated. However, it is clear that psychiatric illnesses or diseases are often composed of overlapping syndromes, which does not mean that the illnesses are comorbid. Rather, it means that each psychiatric illness may manifest itself in a variety of ways, suggesting that an individual could meet criteria for a variety of syndromes. This is particularly true for commonly occurring syndromes such as substance abuse, anxiety, and depression, which may be primary themselves or may, in fact, be secondary to other illnesses. The recognition of this complex presentation of syndromes necessitates some changes in our outlook. The Iowa 500 dealt with rigorously described and defined illnesses. Subsequent studies should be planned in a different fashion, and less clear-cut diagnostic groups should be included as index cases.

There are currently numerous follow-up and family studies of rigorously defined illnesses in anxiety disorders, unipolar and bipolar affective disorders, and schizophrenia. Because of the overlapping syndromes, however, the next methodology may not be to define the study group so rigorously but rather to include patients who, having shown aberrations in behavior and emotion, were directed by the community into some kind of treatment or management. This means that the new study groups will be far more broadly defined, which dictates that new statistical methodologies defining reliable clusters will be developed. Newer data will be accumulated on more rigorously defined premorbid personality characteristics, more specific kinds of genetic transmission, newer laboratory tests, and responses to specific treatments. In the past, we have mainly concerned ourselves with the clinical picture and the course of illness and a roughly defined family history, but now the molecular genetic, neurochemical, and neuropharmacological factors may be coming into the fore and will provide the major points in differential diagnosis and classification. There is considerable reason to be optimistic about progress in these fields. Classification has come a long way from the initial insightful contributions of Kraepelin, and there is no reason why progress cannot continue in a vigorous fashion.

# Appendix I

# The Iowa 500—Bibliography

## 1972

Morrison J, Clancy J, Crowe R, et al: The Iowa 500; I, II: diagnostic validity in mania, depression and schizophrenia. Arch Gen Psychiatry 27:457–461, 1972

## 1973

Clancy J, Crowe R, Winokur G, et al: The Iowa 500:precipitating factors in schizophrenia and primary affective disorder. Compr Psychiatry 14:197–202, 1973

Morrison J, Winokur G, Crowe R, et al: The Iowa 500: the first follow-up. Arch Gen Psychiatry 29:678–682, 1973

Winokur G, Morrison J: The Iowa 500: follow-up of 225 depressives. Br J Psychiatry 123:543–548, 1973

Winokur G, Morrison J, Clancy J: The Iowa 500: familial and clinical finings favor two kinds of depressive illness. Compr Psychiatry 14:99–107, 1973

# 1974

Andreasen NC, Tsuang MT, Canter A: The significance of thought disorder in diagnostic evaluations. Compr Psychiatry 15:27–34, 1974

Clancy J, Tsuang MT, Norton B, et al: The Iowa 500: a comprehensive study of mania, depression and schizophrenia. Journal of the Iowa Medical Society 394–398, 1974

Dempsey GE, Tsuang MT, Struss A, et al: Treatment of schizoaffective disorder. Compr Psychiatry 15:189–197, 1974

Fowler RC, Tsuang MT, Cadoret RJ, et al: A clinical and family comparison of paranoid and non-paranoid schizophrenics. Br J Psychiatry 124:346–351, 1974

Tsuang MT, Fowler R, Cadoret RJ, et al: Schizophrenia among first-degree relatives of paranoid and nonparanoid schizophrenics. Compr Psychiatry 15:295–302, 1974

Tsuang MT, Leaverton PE, Huang KS: Criteria for subtyping poor prognosis schizophrenia: a numerical model for differentiating paranoid from nonparanoid schizophrenia. J Psychiatr Res 10:189–197, 1974

Tsuang MT, Winokur G: Bipolar primary affective disorder. Journal of Operational Psychiatry 6:447–453, 1974

Tsuang MT, Winokur G: Criteria for subtyping schizophrenia: clinical differentiation of hebephrenic and paranoid schizophrenia. Arch Gen Psychiatry 31:43–47, 1974

Winokur G: The division of depressive illness into depression spectrum disease and pure depressive disease. Intl Pharmacopsych 9:5–13, 1974

Winokur G: The use of genetic studies in clarifying clinical issues in schizophrenia, in Biological Mechanisms of Schizophrenia and Schizophrenia: Like Psychoses. Edited by Mitsuda H, Fukuda T. Tokyo, Igaku Shoin, 1974, pp 241–247

Winokur G: Genetic and clinical factors associated with course in depression: contributions to genetic aspects. Pharmakopsychiatrica Neuro Psychopharmakology 7:122–126, 1974

Winokur G, Morrison J, Clancy J: The Iowa 500: clinical and genetic distinction of hebephrenic and paranoid schizophrenia. J Nerv Ment Dis 159:12–19, 1974

# 1975

Fowler RC, Tsuang MT: Spouse of schizophrenics: a blind comparative study. Compr Psychiatry 16:339–342, 1975

Fowler RC, Tsuang MT, Cadoret RJ, et al: Nonpsychotic disorders in the families of process schizophrenics. Acta Psychiatrica Scand 51:153–160, 1975

Tsuang MT: Heterogeneity of schizophrenia. Biol Psychiatry 10:465–474, 1975

Tsuang MT, Winokur G: The Iowa 500: field work in a 35-year follow-up of depression, mania and schizophrenia. Canadian Psychiatric Association Journal 20:359–365, 1975

Tsuang MT, Winokur G: The Iowa 500: preliminary results of field work in a 35 year follow-up of depression, mania and schizophrenia. Canadian Psychiatric Association Journal 20:359–364, 1975

Winokur G: Paranoid vs hebephrenic schizophrenia: clinical and familial (genetic) heterogeneity. Psychopharmacol Comm 1:567–577, 1975

Winokur G: Relationship of genetic factors to course and drug response in schizophrenia, mania and depression, in Genetics and Psychopharmacology: Modern Problems of Pharmacopsychiatry, Vol 20. Edited by Mendlewicz J. Basel, Karger, pp 1–11

Winokur G: The Iowa 500: Heterogeneity and course in manic-depressive illness (bipolar). Compr Psychiatry 16:125–131, 1975

Winokur G, Tsuang MT: A clinical and family history comparison of good outcome and poor outcome schizophrenia. Neuropsychobiology 1:59–64, 1975

Winokur G, Tsuang MT: Elation versus irritability in mania. Compr Psychiatry 16:435–436, 1975

---

# 1976

Fowler RC, Tsuang MT: Schizophrenics' families. Br J Psychiatry 128:100–101, 1976

Tsuang MT, Dempsey GM, Rauscher F: A study of "atypical schizophrenia": comparison with schizophrenia and affective disorder by sex, age of admission, precipitant, outcome and family history. Arch Gen Psychiatry 33:1157–1160, 1976

Winokur G, Tsuang MT: The Iowa 500: suicide in mania, depression, and schizophrenia. Am J Psychiatry 132:650–651, 1976

---

# 1977

Cadoret RJ, Woolson R, Winokur G: The relationship of age of onset in unipolar affective disorder to risk of alcoholism and depression in patients. J Psychiatr Res 13:137–142, 1977

Fowler RC, Tsuang MT, Cadoret RJ: Parental psychiatric illness associated with schizophrenia in the siblings of schizophrenics. Compr Psychiatry 18:271–275, 1977

Fowler RC, Tsuang MT, Cadoret RJ: Psychiatric illness in the offspring of schizophrenics. Compr Psychiatry 18:127–134, 1977

Kathol R, Winokur G: "Organic" and "psychotic" symptoms in unipolar (UP) vs bipolar (BP) depressions. Compr Psychiatry 18:251–253, 1977

Tsuang MT, Dempsey GM, Dvoredsky A, et al: A family history study of schizoaffective disorder. Biol Psychiatry 12:331–338, 1977

Tsuang MT, Winokur G: A combined thirty-five year follow-up and family study of schizophrenia and primary affective disorders: sample selection, methodology of field follow-up, and preliminary mortality rates (paper presented at Society for Life History Research in Psychopathology, Rochester, New York, May 1975), in The Origins and Course of Psychopathology. Edited by Strauss JS, Babigian HM, Roff M. New York, Plenum, 1977, pp 61–78

Tsuang MT, Woolson RF: Mortality in patients with schizophrenia, mania, depression and surgical conditions: a comparison with general population mortality. Br J Psychiatry 130:162–166, 1977

Winokur G: Genetic patterns as they affect psychiatric diagnosis, in Psychiatric Diagnosis. Edited by Rakoff VM, Stancer HC, Kedward HB. New York, Brunner/Mazel, 1977, pp 128–152

Winokur G: Mania and depression: family studies and genetics in relation to treatment, in Psychopharmacology: A Generation of Progress. Edited by Lipton MA, DiMascio A, Killam KF. New York, Raven, 1977, pp 1213–1221

Winokur G, Cadoret R: Genetic studies in depressive disorders, in Handbook of Studies on Depression. Edited by Burrows GD. Amsterdam, Excerpta Medica, 1977, pp 69–71

## 1978

Tsuang MT: Familial subtyping of schizophrenia and affective disorders (paper presented at the Annual Meeting of the American Psychopathological Association, New York, New York, March 1977), in Critical Issues in Psychiatric Diagnosis. Edited by Spitzer RL, Klein DF. New York, Raven, 1978, pp 203–211

Tsuang MT: Suicide in schizophrenics, manics, depressives and surgical controls: a comparison with general population suicide mortality. Arch Gen Psychiatry 35:153–155, 1978

Tsuang MT, Crowe RR, Winokur G, et al: Relatives of schizophrenics, manics, depressives, and controls: an interview
study of 1,331 first-degree relatives (paper presented at the
Second Rochester International Conference on Schizophrenia, Session I: Genetic Transmission, May 3, 1976), in The
Nature of Schizophrenia. Edited by Wynne LC, Cramwell RL,
Matthysse S. New York, Wiley, 1978, pp 52–58
Tsuang MT, Woolson RF: Excess mortality in schizophrenia and
affective disorders: do suicides and accidental deaths solely
account for this excess? Arch Gen Psychiatry 35:1181–1185,
1978
Winokur G: Paranoid versus hebephrenic schizophrenia: a differentiation based on clinical and family (genetic) findings, in
Biochemistry of Mental Disorders: New Vistas, Modern Phar-
macology-Toxicology, Vol 13. Edited by Usdin E, Mandell AJ.
New York, Marcel Dekker, pp 11–29, 1978
Winokur G, Tsuang MT: Expectancy of alcoholism in a U.S. Midwestern population. Journal of Studies on Alcohol 39:1964–
1967, 1978

# 1979

Coryell W, Tsuang MT: Should "non-Feighner" schizophrenia be
classified with affective disorder? J Affect Disord 1:3–8, 1979
Fowler RC, Tsuang MT, Kronfol Z: Communication of suicidal
intent and suicide in unipolar depression: a forty year follow-
up. J Affect Disord 1:219–225, 1979

Tsuang MT: A 35-year follow-up of schizophrenia, mania and depression: an analysis of long-term outcome by marital, employment, institutionalization and psychiatric status (paper presented at the Annual Meeting of the Society of Life History Research in Psychopathology, Fort Worth, Texas, October 6, 1976), in Human Functioning in Longitudinal Perspective: Studies of Normal and Psychopathic Populations. Edited by Sells SB, Crandall R, Roff M, et al. Baltimore, MD, Williams & Wilkins, 1979, pp 46–57

Tsuang MT, Dempsey GM: Long-term outcome of major psychoses, II: "schizoaffective" disorder compared with schizophrenia, affective disorders, and a surgical control group. Arch Gen Psychiatry 36:1302–1304, 1979

Tsuang MT, Dempsey GM, Fleming JA: Can ECT prevent premature death and suicide in "schizoaffective" patients? J Affect Disord 1:167–171, 1979

Tsuang MT, Simpson JC: Le suicide chez les patients atteints de psychose maniaco-depressive, de schizophrenie et d'alcoolism: implications en faveur d'une composante genetique du suicide. Med et Hyg 37:2354–2358, 1979

Tsuang MT, Woolson RF, Fleming JA: Long-term outcome of major psychoses, I: schizophrenia and affective disorders compared with psychiatrically symptom-free surgical conditions. Arch Gen Psychiatry 36:1295–1301, 1979

Winokur G: Familial (genetic) subtypes of pure depressive disease. Am J Psychiatry 136:911–913, 1979

---

## 1980

Quitkin FM, Rifkin A, Tsuang MT, et al: Can schizophrenia with premorbid asociality be genetically distinguished from other forms of schizophrenia? Psychiatr Res 2:99–105, 1980

Tsuang MT: Social effects of schizophrenia and affective disorders: an analysis of marital, residential, occupational, and psychiatric status based on forty-year field follow-up (paper presented at the Triennial Meeting of the World Psychiatric Association Committee on Epidemiology and Community Psychiatry, St. Louis, Missouri, October 18–20, 1980, in The Social Consequences of Psychiatric Illness. Edited by Robins LN, Clayton PJ, Wing JK. New York, Brunner/Mazel, 1980, pp 209–215

Tsuang MT, Winokur G, Crowe RR: Morbidity risks of schizophrenia and affective disorders among first-degree relatives of patients with schizophrenia, mania, depression and surgical conditions. Br J Psychiatry 137:497–504, 1980

Tsuang MT, Woolson RF, Fleming JA: Causes of death in schizophrenia and cancer death. Lancet 1:480–481, 1980

Tsuang MT, Woolson RF, Fleming JA: Causes of death in schizophrenia and manic–depression. Br J Psychiatry 136:239–242, 1980

Tsuang MT, Woolson RF, Fleming JA: Premature death in schizophrenia and affective disorder: an analysis of survival curves and variables affecting the shortened survival. Arch Gen Psychiatry 37:979–983, 1980

Tsuang MT, Woolson RF, Simpson JC: The Iowa Structured Psychiatric Interview: rationale, reliability, and validity. Acta Psychiatr Scand Suppl 62:1–58, 1980

Winokur G: Is there a common genetic factor in bipolar and unipolar affective disorder? Compr Psychiatry 21:460–468, 1980

Woolson RF, Tsuang MT, Fleming JA: Utility of the proportional hazards model in a problem in psychiatry. Journal of Chronic Disease 33:183–195, 1980

Woolson RF, Tsuang MT, Urban LR: Data management in an epidemiological study: experiences from the Iowa 500 field follow-up and family study. Methods Inf Med 19:37–41, 1980

# 1981

Kendler KS, Tsuang MT: The nosology of paranoid schizophrenia and other paranoid psychoses: historical developmental and current status. Schizophr Bull 7:594–610, 1981

Tsuang MT: What is atypical schizophrenia? in Proceedings of the Third Annual Convention of the Japanese Society of Biological Psychiatry, October 23–24, Kyoto, Japan, 1981

Tsuang MT, Woolson RF, Simpson JC: An evaluation of Feighner criteria for schizophrenia and affective disorders using long-term outcome data. Psychology Med 11:281–287, 1981

Tsuang M, Woolson R, Winokur G, et al: Stability of psychiatric diagnosis: schizophrenia and affective disorders followed up over a 30- to 40-year period. Arch Gen Psychiatry 38:535–539, 1981

Winokur G, Tsuang M: Paranoid versus non-paranoid schizophrenia: definition and association, in Biol Psych. Edited by Perris C, Struwe G, Jansson B. Holland, Elsevier/North, 1981, pp 761–765

Winokur G, Tsuang MT, Crowe RR: The Iowa 500: family studies of bipolar and unipolar affective disorders. Psychopharmacol Bull 17:78–80, 1981

Winokur G, Tsuang MT, Crowe RR: The Iowa 500: family studies of unipolar affective disorders. Psychopharmacol Bull 139:78–80, 1981

# 1982

Cadoret R, Winokur G: Genetics and psychiatry, in Clinical Medicine. Edited by Spittell JA Jr. Philadelphia, PA, Harper & Row, 1982, pp 1–7

Coryell W, Tsuang MT: DSM–III schizophreniform disorder: comparison with schizophrenia and affective disorder. Arch Gen Psychiatry 39:66–69, 1982

Coryell W, Tsuang MT: Primary unipolar depression and the prognostic significance of delusions. Arch Gen Psychiatry 39:1181–1184, 1982

Coryell W, Tsuang MT, McDaniel J: Psychiatric features in major depression: is mood congruence important? J Affect Disord 4:227–236, 1982

Pfohl B, Winokur G: The evolution of symptoms in institutionalized hebephrenic/catatonic schizophrenics. Br J Psychiatry 141:567–572, 1982

Tsuang MT: Long-term outcome in schizophrenia. Trends Neurosci 5:203–207, 1982

Tsuang MT: Memory deficit and long–term outcome in schizophrenia: a preliminary study. Psychiatry Res 6:355–360, 1982

Tsuang MT: On research methodology and formulation of diagnostic criteria for "atypical psychosis": a follow–up and family study of "atypical schizophrenia." Japanese Journal of Clinical Psychiatry 11:415–424, 1982

Tsuang MT: Schizophrenia syndromes: the search for subgroups in schizophrenia with brain dysfunction (paper presented at the Fifth Annual Andrew Woods Symposium, "Schizophrenia as a Brain Disease"). Edited by Henn FA, Nasrallah H. New York, Oxford University Press, 1982, pp 14–25

Tsuang MT, Bucher KD, Fleming JA: Testing the monogenic theory of schizophrenia: an application of segregation methods of analysis to blind family study data. Br J Psychiatry 140:595–599, 1982

Winokur G: Depressive illness in late life, in Medical Care for the Elderly. Edited by Smith I. London, SP Medical and Scientific Books, 1982, pp 219–222

Winokur G: The development and validity of familial subtypes in primary unipolar depression. Pharmacopsychiatria 15:142–146, 1982

Winokur G, Tsuang MT, Crowe RR: The Iowa 500: affective disorder in relatives of manic and depressed patients. Am J Psychiatry 139:209–212, 1982

# 1983

Pfohl B, Winokur G: The micropsychopathology of hebephrenic-catatonic schizophrenia. J Nerv Ment Dis 171:296–300, 1983

Tsuang MT: Risk of suicide in the relatives of schizophrenics, manics, depressives, and controls. J Clin Psychiatry 44:396–400, 1983

Tsuang MT, Bucher KD, Fleming JA: A search for "schizophrenia spectrum disorders": an application of the multiple threshold model to blind family study data. Br J Psychiatry 143:572–577, 1983

Winokur G: Controversies in depression, or do clinicians know something after all? in Treatment of Depression: Old Controversies and New Approaches. Edited by Clayton P, Barrett J. New York, Raven, 1983, pp 153–168

Winokur G, Crowe R: Bipolar illness: the sex-polarity effect in affectively ill family members. Arch Gen Psychiatry 40:57–58, 1983

# 1984

Kendler KS, Gruenberg AM, Tsuang MT: Outcome of schizophrenia subtypes defined by four diagnostic systems. Arch Gen Psychiatry 41:149–154, 1984

Kronfol Z, Turner R, Nasrallah H, et al: Leukocyte regulation in depression and schizophrenia. Psychiatry Res 13:13–18, 1984

Tsuang MT, Simpson JC: Schizoaffective disorder: concept and reality. Schizophr Bull 10:14–25, 1984

Tsuang MT, Winokur G, Crowe RR: Psychiatric disorders among relatives of surgical controls. J Clin Psychiatry 45:420–422, 1984

Winokur G: Psychosis in bipolar and unipolar affective illness with special reference to schizoaffective disorder. Br J Psychiatry 145:236–242, 1984

---

# 1985

Coryell W, Tsuang MT: Major depression with mood-congruent or mood incongruent psychotic features: outcome after 40 years. Am J Psychiatry 142:479–482, 1985

Kendler KS, Gruenberg AM, Tsuang MT: Psychiatric illness in first degree relatives of schizophrenic and surgical control patients: a family study using DSM-III criteria. Arch Gen Psychiatry 42:770–779, 1985

Kendler KS, Gruenberg AM, Tsuang MT: Subtype stability in schizophrenia. Am J Psychiatry 142:827–832, 1985

Loyd DW, Simpson JC, Tsuang MT: A family study of sex differences in the diagnosis of atypical schizophrenia. Am J Psychiatry 142:1366–1368, 1985

Loyd DW, Simpson JC, Tsuang MT: Are there sex differences in the long-term outcome of schizophrenia? comparisons with mania, depression, and surgical controls. J Nerv Ment Dis 171:543–649, 1985

Tsuang MT, Bucher KD, Fleming JA, et al: Transmission of affective disorders: an application of segregation analysis to blind family study data. J Psychiatry Res 19:23–29, 1985

Tsuang MT, Faraone SV, Fleming JA: Familial transmission of major affective disorders: is there evidence supporting the distinction between unipolar and bipolar disorders? Br J Psychiatry 146:268–271, 1985

Tsuang MT, Kendler KS, Gruenberg AM: A blind family study of DSM-III schizophrenia (paper presented at the Annual Meeting of the International Conference IV, Kobe Japan, November 1983), in Genetic Aspects of Human Behavior. Edited by Sakai T, Tsuboi T. Tokyo, Igaku Shoin, 1985, pp 57–61

Tsuang MT, Kendler KS, Gruenberg AM: DSM–III schizophrenia: is there evidence for familial transmission? Acta Psychiatr Scand 71:77–83, 1985

Tsuang MT, Simpson JC: Mortality studies in psychiatry. Arch Gen Psychiatry 42:98–103, 1985

Winokur G: Comparative studies of familial psychopathology in affective disorders, in Genetic Aspects of Human Behavior. Edited by Sakai T, Tsuboi T. Tokyo, Aino Hospital Foundation Igaku Shoin, 1985, pp 87–96

Winokur G: Familial psychopathology in delusional disorder. Compr Psychiatry 26:241–248, 1985

## 1986

Coryell W, Tsuang MT: Outcome after forty years in DSM-III schizophreniform disorder. Arch Gen Psychiatry 43:324–328, 1986

Kendler KS, Gruenberg AM, Tsuang MT: A DSM–III family study of the non-schizophrenic psychotic disorders. Am J Psychiatry 143:1098–1105, 1986

Kronfol Z, Turner R, House D, et al: Elevated blood neutrophil concentration in mania. J Clin Psychiatry 47:63–65, 1986

Simpson JC, Woolson RF, Tsuang MT: Computation of expected deaths for prediction and for long-term follow-up studies. Methods Inf Med 25:165–170, 1986

Tsuang MT, Fleming JA: Long-term outcome of schizophrenia and other psychoses, in The Proceeding of Symposium, University of Heidelberg, Search for the Causes of Schizophrenia, September 24–26, 1986, pp 88–97

Tsuang MT, Simpson JC, Fleming JA: Diagnostic criteria for subtyping schizoaffective disorder, in Schizoaffective Psychosis. Edited by Marneros A, Tsuang MT. Berlin-Heidelberg, Springer-Verlag, 1986, pp 50–59

Tsuang M, Winokur G, Crowe R: Morbidity risks of schizophrenia and affective disorders among first degree relatives of patients with schizophrenia, mania, depression, and surgical conditions, in Contemporary Issues in Schizophrenia. Edited by Kerr A, Snaith P, Gaskell. London, Royal College of Psychiatrists, 1986

Winokur G: Classification of chronic psychoses including delusional disorders and schizophrenias. Psychopathology 19:30–34, 1986

Winokur G, Dennert J, Angst J: Independent familial transmission of psychotic symptomatology in the affective disorders or does delusional depression breed true? Psych Fenn 17, 1986

---

# 1987

Faraone SV, Lyons MJ, Tsuang MT: Sex differences in affective disorder: genetic transmission. Genet Epidemiol 4:331–343, 1987

Kendler KS, Tsuang MT, Hays P: Age of onset in schizophrenia: a familial perspective. Arch Gen Psychiatry 44:881–890, 1987

Loyd DW, Tsuang MT: Schizoaffective disorder and depression associated with psychosis, in Presentations of Depression. Edited by Cameron CG. 1987, pp 67–82

Tsuang MT: Long-term follow-up of the major psychoses (paper presented at the Second Pacific Congress of Psychiatry, Manila, Philippines, May 12–16, 1980), in Longitudinal Research in the United States. Edited by Mednick SA, Harway M, Finelo KM, Praeger, 1987, pp 403–409

Tsuang MT: Predictors of poor and good outcome in schizophrenia, in Conference Book From the November 1979 Society for Life History Research in Psychopathology and Society for the Study of Social Biology Meeting. Edited by Erlenmeyer-Kimling L, Miller N. Lawrence Erlbaum, 1987, pp 195–203

Winokur G, Pfohl B, Tsuang MT: A 30–40 year follow-up of he-bephrenic catatonic schizophrenia, in International Conference on Schizophrenia and Aging. Edited by Miller N. New York, Guilford, 1987, pp 53–60

Winokur G, Wesner R: From unipolar depression to bipolar illness: 29 who changed. Acta Psychiatrica Scand 76:59–63, 1987

## 1988

Buda M, Tsuang MT, Fleming JA: Causes of death in DSM–III schizophrenics and other psychotics NEC (atypical group): a comparison with the general population. Arch Gen Psychiatry 45:283–285, 1988

Faraone SV, Tsuang MT: Familial links between schizophrenia and other disorders: application of the multifactorial poly-genic model. Psychiat: Interpers Biolog Process 51:37–47, 1988

Kendler KS, Gruenberg AM, Tsuang MT: A family study of the subtypes of schizophrenia. Am J Psychiatry 145:57–62, 1988

Kendler KS, Tsuang MT: Outcome and familial psychopathology in schizophrenia. Arch Gen Psychiatry 45:338–346, 1988

Rogers K, Winokur G: The genetics of schizoaffective disorder and the schizophrenia spectrum, in Handbook of Schizophrenia: Nosology, Epidemiology and Genetics of Schizophrenia. Edited by Tsuang M, Simpson J. Amsterdam, Elsevier, 1988, pp 481–500

Tsuang MT, Fleming JA, Kendler KS, et al: Selection of controls for family studies: biases and implications. Arch Gen Psychiatry 45:1006–1008, 1988

## 1989

Goldstein JM, Tsuang MT, Faraone SV: Gender and schizophrenia: implications for understanding the heterogeneity of the illness. Psychiatr Res 28:243–253, 1989

## 1990

Faraone SV, Kremen WS, Tsuang MT: The genetic transmission of major affective disorders: mathematical models and linkage analysis. Psychol Bull 108:109–127, 1990

Goldstein JM, Faraone SV, Chen W, et al: Sex differences in the familial transmission of schizophrenia. Br J Psychiatry 156:819–826, 1990

Goldstein JM, Santangelo SL, Simpson JC, et al: The role of gender in identifying subtypes of schizophrenia: a latent class analytic approach. Schizophr Bull 16:263–275, 1990

Goldstein JM, Tsuang MT: Gender and schizophrenia: an introduction and synthesis of findings. Schizophr Bull 16:179–183, 1990

Rogers K, Winokur G: Diagnostic separateness of schizophrenia and affective disorder, in Depression in Schizophrenia. Edited by Delisi L. Washington, DC, American Psychiatric Press, 1990, pp 61–77

Tsuang MT: Follow-up studies of schizoaffective disorders: a comparison with affective disorders, in Affective and Schizoaffective Disorders: Similarities and Differences. Edited by Marneros A, Tsuang MT. Berlin-Heidelberg, Springer-Verlag, 1990, pp 123–129

Tsuang MT: The heterogeneity of schizoaffective disorders, in Affective and Schizoaffective Disorders: Similarities and Differences. Edited by Marneros A, Tsuang MT. Berlin-Heidelberg, Springer-Verlag, 1990, pp 274–276

Tsuang MT, Lyons MJ, Faraone SV: Heterogeneity of schizo-phrenia: conceptual models and analytic strategies. Br J Psychiatry 156:17–26, 1990

## 1991

Goldstein JM, Faraone SV, Chen WJ, et al: Gender differences in the familial transmission of schizophrenia. Schizophr Res 4:258–259, 1991

Tsuang MT: Morbidity risks of schizophrenia and affective disorders among first-degree relatives of patients with schizoaffective disorder. Br J Psychiatry 158:165–170, 1991

Tsuang MT, Gilbertson MW, Faraone SV: The genetics of schizophrenia: current knowledge and future directions. Schizophr Res 4:157–171, 1991

Winokur G: Mania and Depression: A Classification of Syndrome and Disease. Baltimore, MD, Johns Hopkins University Press, 1991

Winokur G, Coryell W: A case for discontinuity in the psychotic illnesses, in Biological Psychiatry. Edited by Racagni G, Brunello N, Fukuda T. Amsterdam, Elsevier, 1991, pp 506–509

## 1992

Tsuang MT, Hsieh C, Fleming JA: Group comparison approaches in psychiatric research, in Research in Psychiatry: Issues, Strategies, and Methods. Edited by Hsu, Hersen. New York, Plenum, 1992, pp 107–132

Winokur G: A familial ("genetic") methodology for determining valid types of affective illnesses. Pharmacopsychiatry 25:14–17, 1992

## In Press

Chen WJ, Faraone SV, Tsuang MT: Linkage studies of schizophrenia: a simulation study of statistical power. Genet Epidemiol (in press)

Goldstein JM, Faraone SV, Chen WJ, Tsuang MT: Gender and the familial risk for schizophrenia: disentangling confounding factors. Schizophr Res (in press)

# Appendix II

# Code Book—Index Admission and Chart Follow-Up for the Iowa 500 Study

Following are the original data recorded from the charts. Items 1–3 were identifying numbers, and items 4–95 contain demographic data, family history, and follow-up data. Originally, there were 200 schizophrenic patients who were entered into the study, 100 bipolar, and 225 unipolar patients. A word should be said about the unipolar and bipolar patients. Of the 225 unipolar patients, 22 became bipolar in either the follow-up chart or fieldwork. As a consequence, the bipolar group, which started with 100 patients, totals 122 in the assessment presented in this Appendix. The unipolar group is reduced to 203.

## Code Book

### *Index Admission and Chart Follow-Up*

| 1–3. Code Numbers | S | B | U |
|---|---|---|---|
| **4.　Sex** | | | |
| 0.　Female | 98 | 68 | 118 |
| 1.　Male | 102 | 54 | 85 |
| **5.　Age at Admission** | | | |
| 1.　10–19 | 19 | 16 | 1 |
| 2.　20–29 | 101 | 39 | 26 |
| 3.　30–39 | 64 | 22 | 37 |
| 4.　40–49 | 11 | 19 | 63 |
| 5.　50–59 | 4 | 24 | 63 |
| 6.　60–69 | 1 | 2 | 13 |
| **6.　Diagnosis, Ours** | | | |
| 0.　Unipolar depressive | 0 | 22 | 203 |
| 1.　Bipolar depressive (had mania before) | 0 | 6 | 0 |
| 2.　Unipolar manic | 0 | 55 | 0 |
| 3.　Bipolar manic (had depression before) | 0 | 31 | 0 |
| 4.　Mixed manic depressive | 0 | 7 | 0 |
| 5.　Circular during admission | 0 | 1 | 0 |
| 6.　Schizophrenic, paranoid | 62 | 0 | 0 |
| 7.　Schizophrenic, hebephrenic | 115 | 0 | 0 |
| 8.　Schizophrenic, catatonic | 15 | 0 | 0 |
| 9.　Schizophrenic, uncertain type | 8 | 0 | 0 |
| **7.　Age at Onset of First Illness** | | | |
| 0.　Unknown | 1 | 1 | 1 |
| 1.　10–19 | 42 | 33 | 10 |
| 2.　20–29 | 114 | 37 | 54 |
| 3.　30–39 | 39 | 19 | 48 |
| 4.　40–49 | 4 | 15 | 46 |
| 5.　50–59 | 0 | 16 | 37 |
| 6.　60–69 | 0 | 1 | 7 |

*Note.* S = schizophrenic; B = bipolar; U = unipolar.

| 8. | Previous Hospital Admissions | | | |
|----|------------------------------|-----|-----|-----|
| 0. | None | 154 | 76 | 173 |
| 1. | 1 | 32 | 29 | 19 |
| 2. | 2 | 10 | 12 | 7 |
| 3. | 3 | 4 | 2 | 3 |
| 4. | 4 | 0 | 1 | 1 |
| 5. | 5 | 0 | 1 | 0 |
| 6. | 6 | 0 | 0 | 0 |
| 7. | 7 | 0 | 0 | 0 |
| 8. | 8 | 0 | 1 | 0 |

| 9. | Subsequent Inpatient Admissions | | | |
|----|---------------------------------|-----|-----|-----|
| 0. | None | 183 | 100 | 185 |
| 1. | 1 | 14 | 17 | 10 |
| 2. | 2 | 2 | 4 | 5 |
| 3. | 3 | 0 | 1 | 1 |
| 4. | 4 | 0 | 0 | 0 |
| 5. | 5 | 1 | 0 | 1 |
| 6. | 6 | 0 | 0 | 1 |

| 10. | Discharged to: | | | |
|-----|----------------|-----|-----|-----|
| 0. | Community (including home, self, relative, etc.) | 53 | 49 | 99 |
| 1. | State hospital | 109 | 46 | 72 |
| 2. | Other hospital | 11 | 17 | 12 |
| 3. | Discharged to community AMA | 27 | 10 | 20 |

| 11. | Length of Illness at Index Admission | | | |
|-----|--------------------------------------|-----|-----|-----|
| 0. | 2 Weeks | 0 | 22 | 0 |
| 1. | 1 Month | 2 | 46 | 24 |
| 2. | 3 Months | 0 | 18 | 66 |
| 3. | 6 Months | 29 | 22 | 58 |
| 4. | 1 Year | 31 | 5 | 34 |
| 5. | 2 Years | 35 | 7 | 13 |
| 6. | 3 Years | 36 | 0 | 4 |
| 7. | 5 Years | 34 | 1 | 4 |
| 8. | 10 Years or more | 32 | 1 | 0 |
| 9. | Unknown | 1 | 0 | 0 |

| 12. | **Dysphoria** | | | |
|-----|------------|-----|-----|-----|
| 0. | Absent | 192 | 73 | 0 |
| 1. | Depressed (or synonymous) only | 5 | 18 | 48 |
| 2. | Fearful | 1 | 0 | 0 |
| 3. | Worried | 0 | 1 | 1 |
| 4. | Depressed and irritable | 1 | 4 | 7 |
| 5. | Depressed and fearful | 0 | 6 | 16 |
| 6. | Depressed and worried | 0 | 15 | 98 |
| 7. | Depressed and more than one other | 1 | 3 | 33 |
| 8. | Not depressed but two or more others | 0 | 2 | 0 |
| 13. | **Anorexia** | | | |
| 0. | No | 160 | 53 | 20 |
| 1. | Yes | 32 | 50 | 152 |
| 2. | Unknown | 8 | 19 | 31 |
| 14. | **Weight Loss (2 lb/wk or 10 or more per year)** | | | |
| 0. | No | 173 | 62 | 40 |
| 1. | Yes | 13 | 22 | 78 |
| 2. | Unknown | 14 | 38 | 85 |
| 15. | **Sleep Difficulty** | | | |
| 0. | None | 136 | 14 | 8 |
| 1. | Early A.M. awakening | 3 | 9 | 29 |
| 2. | Other sleep difficulty (decreased) | 41 | 74 | 137 |
| 3. | Hypersomnia | 5 | 0 | 1 |
| 4. | Early A.M. awakening and other sleep difficulty (decreased) | 0 | 10 | 4 |
| 5. | Early A.M. awakening and hypersomnia | 1 | 0 | 0 |
| 6. | Other sleep difficulty | 0 | 0 | 0 |
| 7. | All three | 0 | 0 | 0 |
| 8. | Sleep trouble but uncertain what kind | 8 | 6 | 19 |
| 9. | Unknown if sleep difficulty | 6 | 9 | 5 |
| 16. | **Loss of Energy (easily fatigued, tiredness)** | | | |
| 0. | No | 150 | 89 | 37 |
| 1. | Yes | 46 | 28 | 140 |
| 2. | Unknown | 4 | 5 | 26 |

**17. Agitation**

| | | | | |
|---|---|---|---|---|
| 0. | No | 155 | 56 | 57 |
| 1. | Yes | 44 | 66 | 145 |
| 2. | Unknown | 1 | 0 | 1 |

**18. Retardation**

| | | | | |
|---|---|---|---|---|
| 0. | No | 191 | 96 | 81 |
| 1. | Yes | 8 | 26 | 121 |
| 2. | Unknown | 1 | 0 | 1 |

**19. Loss of Interest in Usual Activities**

| | | | | |
|---|---|---|---|---|
| 0. | No | 91 | 81 | 14 |
| 1. | Yes | 106 | 34 | 177 |
| 2. | Unknown | 3 | 7 | 12 |

**20. Sex Drive**

| | | | | |
|---|---|---|---|---|
| 0. | Decreased | 53 | 19 | 45 |
| 1. | Increased | 20 | 33 | 7 |
| 2. | Unknown | 127 | 70 | 151 |

**21. Feelings of Self-Reproach or Guilt, Worthlessness, Sinfulness, Failure**

| | | | | |
|---|---|---|---|---|
| 0. | No | 184 | 88 | 67 |
| 1. | Yes | 12 | 29 | 123 |
| 2. | Delusional | 2 | 4 | 11 |
| 3. | Unknown | 2 | 1 | 2 |

**22. Thinking Difficulty (trouble thinking, concentrating, slow, mixed-up)**

| | | | | |
|---|---|---|---|---|
| 0. | No | 133 | 60 | 82 |
| 1. | Yes | 67 | 60 | 111 |
| 2. | Unknown | 0 | 2 | 10 |

**23. Suicide**

| | | | | |
|---|---|---|---|---|
| 0. | None of below at any time | 182 | 90 | 55 |
| 1. | Suicide attempt, present illness (PI) | 4 | 8 | 57 |
| 2. | Suicide attempt, PI and in past | 0 | 0 | 0 |
| 3. | Suicide attempt in past, not PI | 1 | 3 | 2 |
| 4. | Suicidal thoughts, PI, no attempts ever | 13 | 21 | 87 |

| | | | | |
|---|---|---|---|---|
| 5. | Suicidal thoughts, P.I., past suicide attempt | 0 | 0 | 2 |

**24. Increased Tearfulness**

| | | | | |
|---|---|---|---|---|
| 0. | No | 155 | 70 | 66 |
| 1. | Yes | 45 | 50 | 135 |
| 2. | Unknown | 0 | 2 | 2 |

**25. Diurnal Variation**

| | | | | |
|---|---|---|---|---|
| 0. | No | 177 | 37 | 37 |
| 1. | Yes | 1 | 8 | 38 |
| 2. | Unknown | 22 | 77 | 128 |

**26. Euphoric (too happy, powerful, owns the whole world), Irritable**

| | | | | |
|---|---|---|---|---|
| 0. | None | 196 | 28 | 203 |
| 1. | Euphoric | 4 | 28 | 0 |
| 2. | Irritable | 0 | 8 | 0 |
| 3. | Euphoric and irritable | 0 | 58 | 0 |

**27. Hyperactivity (motor, social, or sexual)**

| | | | | |
|---|---|---|---|---|
| 0. | No | 191 | 29 | 199 |
| 1. | Yes | 9 | 93 | 4 |

**28. Pressure of Speech (or pressure to keep talking)**

| | | | | |
|---|---|---|---|---|
| 0. | No | 193 | 29 | 200 |
| 1. | Yes | 7 | 92 | 3 |
| 2. | Unknown | 0 | 1 | 0 |

**29. Flight of Ideas (or racing thoughts)**

| | | | | |
|---|---|---|---|---|
| 0. | No | 198 | 43 | 203 |
| 1. | Yes | 2 | 77 | 0 |
| 2. | Unknown | 0 | 2 | 0 |

**30. Grandiosity**

| | | | | |
|---|---|---|---|---|
| 0. | No | 173 | 80 | 203 |
| 1. | Yes | 7 | 24 | 0 |
| 2. | Yes and delusional | 20 | 17 | 0 |
| 3. | Unknown | 0 | 1 | 0 |

**31. Distractible**

| | | | | |
|---|---|---|---|---|
| 0. | No | 121 | 35 | 172 |
| 1. | Yes | 76 | 84 | 19 |
| 2. | Unknown | 3 | 3 | 12 |

| 32. | Excessive or Inappropriate Spending | | | |
|-----|-------------------------------------|-----|-----|-----|
| 0. | No | 197 | 100 | 202 |
| 1. | Yes | 3 | 19 | 1 |
| 2. | Unknown | 0 | 3 | 0 |

| 33. | Marital status (at time of admission) | | | |
|-----|---------------------------------------|-----|-----|-----|
| 0. | Unknown | 0 | 0 | 1 |
| 1. | Married | 40 | 69 | 149 |
| 2. | Single | 151 | 45 | 35 |
| 3. | Divorced | 5 | 3 | 5 |
| 4. | Separated | 3 | 1 | 4 |
| 5. | Widowed | 1 | 4 | 9 |

| 34. | Poor Premorbid Social Adjustment or Work History | | | |
|-----|--------------------------------------------------|-----|-----|-----|
| 0. | No | 99 | 117 | 194 |
| 1. | Yes | 100 | 4 | 7 |
| 2. | Unknown | 1 | 1 | 2 |

| 35. | Passivity (including influenced in unusual ways) | | | |
|-----|--------------------------------------------------|-----|-----|-----|
| 0. | No | 115 | 117 | 198 |
| 1. | Yes | 80 | 5 | 5 |
| 2. | Unknown | 5 | 0 | 0 |

| 36. | Depersonalization or Derealization | | | |
|-----|------------------------------------|-----|-----|-----|
| 0. | No | 159 | 115 | 186 |
| 1. | Yes | 33 | 7 | 17 |
| 2. | Unknown | 8 | 0 | 0 |

| 37. | Number of Previous Episodes of Illness | | | |
|-----|----------------------------------------|-----|-----|-----|
| 0. | None | 193 | 59 | 114 |
| 1. | 1 | 6 | 34 | 59 |
| 2. | 2 | 1 | 10 | 20 |
| 3. | 3 | 0 | 6 | 4 |
| 4. | 4 | 0 | 5 | 4 |
| 5. | 5 | 0 | 2 | 0 |
| 6. | 6 | 0 | 1 | 1 |
| 7. | 7 | 0 | 0 | 0 |
| 8. | 8 | 0 | 4 | 1 |
| 9. | Unknown | 0 | 1 | 0 |

| 38. | Changed Perception | | | |
|---|---|---|---|---|
| 0. | No | 136 | 109 | 183 |
| 1. | Yes | 56 | 13 | 20 |
| 2. | Unknown | 8 | 0 | 0 |

| 39. | Symbolism (primary delusions) | | | |
|---|---|---|---|---|
| 0. | No | 143 | 118 | 195 |
| 1. | Yes | 50 | 4 | 8 |
| 2. Unknown | | 7 | 0 | 0 |

| 40. | Persecutory Delusions, Being Followed, Spied Upon, Tampered With, Thought Broadcasting, etc. | | | |
|---|---|---|---|---|
| 0. | Neither | 21 | 56 | 100 |
| 1. | Persecutory delusions | 83 | 30 | 30 |
| 2. | Thought broadcasting | 0 | 0 | 1 |
| 3. | Both | 12 | 1 | 0 |
| 4. | Unknown | 4 | 0 | 1 |
| 5. | Other delusions | 22 | 26 | 49 |
| 6. | Persecutory and other delusions | 52 | 8 | 22 |
| 7. | Thought broadcasting and other delusions | 0 | 0 | 0 |
| 8. | All three types of delusions | 6 | 1 | 0 |

| 41. | Auditory Hallucinations (significant) | | | |
|---|---|---|---|---|
| 0. | No | 88 | 105 | 190 |
| 1. | Yes | 108 | 17 | 12 |
| 2. | Unknown | 4 | 0 | 1 |

| 42. | Visual Hallucinations | | | |
|---|---|---|---|---|
| 0. | No | 139 | 111 | 200 |
| 1. | Yes | 52 | 11 | 3 |
| 2. | Unknown | 9 | 0 | 0 |

| 43. | Haptic Hallucinations (tactile or genital) | | | |
|---|---|---|---|---|
| 0. | No | 130 | 115 | 188 |
| 1. | Yes | 58 | 7 | 15 |
| 2. | Unknown | 12 | 0 | 0 |

| 44. | Blocking, Mute | | | |
|---|---|---|---|---|
| 0. | None | 86 | 119 | 197 |
| 1. | Mute | 6 | 1 | 6 |

| | | | | |
|---|---|---|---|---|
| 2. | Blocking | 15 | 1 | 0 |
| 3. | Tangential | 61 | 1 | 0 |
| 4. | Blocking and tangential | 24 | 0 | 0 |
| 5. | Blocking and mute | 0 | 0 | 0 |
| 6. | Tangential and mute | 4 | 0 | 0 |
| 7. | All three | 4 | 0 | 0 |

**45. Motor Symptoms (tics, grimaces, waxy flexibility, postures, stereotypes, verbigeration) that is, Catatonic Symptoms**

| | | | | |
|---|---|---|---|---|
| 0. | No | 136 | 110 | 199 |
| 1. | Yes | 63 | 12 | 4 |
| 2. | Unknown | 1 | 0 | 0 |

**46. Affect**

| | | | | |
|---|---|---|---|---|
| 1. | Flat or blunt | 19 | 117 | 203 |
| 2. | Inappropriate | 144 | 1 | 0 |
| 3. | Unknown | 37 | 4 | 0 |

**47. Anxiety Attacks**

| | | | | |
|---|---|---|---|---|
| 0. | No | 200 | 120 | 191 |
| 1. | Yes | 0 | 2 | 9 |
| 2. | Unknown | 0 | 0 | 3 |

**48. Many Somatic Complaints During Life**

| | | | | |
|---|---|---|---|---|
| 0. | No | 177 | 115 | 189 |
| 1. | Yes | 20 | 4 | 7 |
| 2. | Unknown | 3 | 3 | 7 |

**49. Phobias**

| | | | | |
|---|---|---|---|---|
| 0. | No | 193 | 119 | 192 |
| 1. | Yes | 1 | 0 | 3 |
| 2. | Yes in past | 1 | 0 | 0 |
| 3. | Yes in past and now | 0 | 0 | 1 |
| 4. | Unknown | 5 | 3 | 7 |

**50. Obsessions and/or Compulsions**

| | | | | |
|---|---|---|---|---|
| 0. | No | 191 | 118 | 190 |
| 1. | Yes | 5 | 2 | 4 |
| 2. | Yes in past | 0 | 0 | 0 |
| 3. | Yes in past and now | 1 | 0 | 1 |
| 4. | Unknown | 3 | 2 | 8 |

| 51. | **Social Withdrawal, Seclusiveness** | | | |
|-----|---------------------------------------|-----|-----|-----|
| 0. | No | 56 | 108 | 129 |
| 1. | Yes | 144 | 12 | 64 |
| 2. | Unknown | 0 | 2 | 10 |

| 52. | **Any Memory Deficit, Disorientation (during hospital stay)** | | | |
|-----|----------------------------------------------------------------|-----|-----|-----|
| 0. | No | 175 | 106 | 181 |
| 1. | Yes | 22 | 15 | 20 |
| 2. | Unknown | 3 | 1 | 2 |

| 53. | **Antisocial Behavior (including marked school difficulties)** | | | |
|-----|----------------------------------------------------------------|-----|-----|-----|
| 1. | Yes | 185 | 120 | 202 |
| 2. | Unknown | 15 | 2 | 1 |

| 54. | **Age Father Disappeared From Observation (death, alive, or last admission of proband)** | | | |
|-----|-------------------------------------------------------------------------------------------|-----|-----|-----|
| 0. | Unknown | 0 | 3 | 3 |
| 1. | 10–19 | 0 | 0 | 0 |
| 2. | 20–29 | 2 | 1 | 3 |
| 3. | 30–39 | 15 | 5 | 17 |
| 4. | 40–49 | 32 | 14 | 18 |
| 5. | 50–59 | 70 | 39 | 35 |
| 6. | 60–69 | 53 | 24 | 43 |
| 7. | 70–79 | 23 | 21 | 59 |
| 8. | 80–89 | 5 | 15 | 24 |
| 9. | 90– | 0 | 0 | 1 |

| 55. | **Dx Father** | | | |
|-----|---------------|-----|-----|-----|
| 0. | Not noted | 128 | 81 | 133 |
| 1. | Bipolar psychosis | 1 | 1 | 1 |
| 2. | Depressive illness | 4 | 8 | 12 |
| 3. | Some kind of affective disorder (remitting) | 3 | 1 | 7 |
| 4. | Schizophrenia, paranoid type | 0 | 0 | 1 |
| 5. | Schizophrenia, other or unknown type | 1 | 1 | 0 |
| 6. | Alcoholism | 23 | 10 | 23 |
| 7. | Unknown psychiatric illness (psychotic) | | | |

| 8. | Unknown psychiatric illness, minor (neurosis, personality, etc.) | 4 | 4 | 5 |
| 9. | Father unknown | 36 | 15 | 19 |

**56. Father**

| 1. | Chronic hospitalization | 0 | 3 | 6 |
| 2. | Hospitalized and discharged | 5 | 4 | 3 |
| 3. | Saw a psychiatrist, OPD | 0 | 0 | 0 |
| 4. | Saw a physician for psychiatric illness | 0 | 0 | 0 |
| 5. | Seen in social agency | 3 | 0 | 0 |
| 6. | Suicide (takes precedence) | 5 | 2 | 13 |
| 7. | None of the above | 172 | 100 | 162 |
| 8. | Unknown | 15 | 13 | 19 |

**57. Age Mother Disappeared From Observation (death, alive, or last admission of proband)**

| 0. | Unknown | 0 | 2 | 3 |
| 1. | 10–19 | 0 | 0 | 0 |
| 2. | 20–29 | 7 | 3 | 4 |
| 3. | 30–39 | 9 | 9 | 11 |
| 4. | 40–49 | 41 | 17 | 13 |
| 5. | 50–59 | 78 | 41 | 38 |
| 6. | 60–69 | 45 | 27 | 53 |
| 7. | 70–79 | 16 | 17 | 57 |
| 8. | 80–89 | 4 | 6 | 21 |
| 9. | 90– | 0 | 0 | 3 |

**58. Dx Mother**

| 0. | Not noted | 136 | 93 | 158 |
| 1. | Bipolar psychosis | 2 | 1 | 0 |
| 2. | Depressive illness | 6 | 2 | 11 |
| 3. | Some kind of affective disorder (remitting) | 4 | 7 | 9 |
| 4. | Schizophrenia, paranoid type | 3 | 0 | 0 |
| 5. | Schizophrenia, other or unknown type | 3 | 0 | 0 |
| 6. | Alcoholism | 0 | 0 | 0 |
| 7. | Unknown psychiatric illness (psychotic) | 3 | 3 | 2 |

| 8. | Unknown psychiatric illness, minor (e.g., neurosis, personality disorder) | 43 | 15 | 22 |
|----|----|----|----|----|
| 9. | Mother unknown | 0 | 1 | 1 |

| 59. | **Mother** | | | |
|----|----|----|----|----|
| 1. | Chronic hospitalization | 2 | 1 | 2 |
| 2. | Hospitalized and discharged | 5 | 6 | 6 |
| 3. | Saw a psychiatrist, OPD | 1 | 0 | 1 |
| 4. | Saw a physician for psychiatric illness | 2 | 0 | 2 |
| 5. | Seen in social agency | 0 | 0 | 0 |
| 6. | Suicide (takes precedence) | 0 | 1 | 2 |
| 7. | None of the above | 180 | 105 | 178 |
| 8. | Unknown | 10 | 9 | 12 |

| 60. | **Number of Brothers 15+** | | | |
|----|----|----|----|----|
| 0. | None | 58 | 18 | 34 |
| 1. | 1 | 58 | 41 | 40 |
| 2. | 2 | 40 | 26 | 48 |
| 3. | 3 | 18 | 14 | 43 |
| 4. | 4 | 17 | 12 | 14 |
| 5. | 5 | 5 | 6 | 12 |
| 6. | 6 | 2 | 1 | 10 |
| 7. | 7 | 0 | 0 | 2 |
| 8. | 8 or more | 1 | 1 | 0 |
| 9. | Unknown | 1 | 3 | 0 |

| 61. | **Number of Sisters 15+** | | | |
|----|----|----|----|----|
| 0. | None | 47 | 22 | 38 |
| 1. | 1 | 70 | 34 | 54 |
| 2. | 2 | 41 | 31 | 41 |
| 3. | 3 | 19 | 14 | 30 |
| 4. | 4 | 12 | 11 | 18 |
| 5. | 5 | 6 | 4 | 14 |
| 6. | 6 | 3 | 1 | 6 |
| 7. | 7 | 1 | 2 | 2 |
| 8. | 8 or more | 0 | 0 | 0 |
| 9. | Unknown | 1 | 3 | 0 |

| 62. | **Number of Brothers affective disorder (AD) (remitting illness)** | | | |
|----|----|----|----|----|
| 0. | None | 194 | 106 | 173 |
| 1. | 1 | 4 | 12 | 22 |

| | | | | |
|---|---|---|---|---|
| 2. | 2 | 1 | 1 | 5 |
| 3. | 3 | 0 | 0 | 0 |
| 4. | 4 | 0 | 0 | 1 |
| 5. | 5 | 0 | 0 | 0 |
| 6. | 6 | 0 | 0 | 0 |
| 7. | 7 | 0 | 0 | 0 |
| 8. | 8 | 0 | 0 | 0 |
| 9. | Unknown | 1 | 3 | 2 |

**63. Number of Sisters AD (remitting illness)**

| | | | | |
|---|---|---|---|---|
| 0. | None | 192 | 106 | 167 |
| 1. | 1 | 6 | 12 | 32 |
| 2. | 2 | 0 | 0 | 3 |
| 3. | 3 | 0 | 0 | 0 |
| 4. | 4 | 0 | 0 | 0 |
| 5. | 5 | 0 | 0 | 0 |
| 6. | 6 | 0 | 0 | 0 |
| 7. | 7 | 0 | 0 | 0 |
| 8. | 8 | 0 | 0 | 0 |
| 9. | Unknown | 2 | 4 | 1 |

**64. Number of Brothers Schizophrenic (deteriorating illness)**

| | | | | |
|---|---|---|---|---|
| 0. | None | 195 | 116 | 198 |
| 1. | 1 | 2 | 2 | 3 |
| 2. | 2 | 0 | 1 | 0 |
| 3. | 3 | 0 | 0 | 0 |
| 4. | 4 | 0 | 0 | 0 |
| 5. | 5 | 0 | 0 | 0 |
| 6. | 6 | 0 | 0 | 0 |
| 7. | 7 | 0 | 0 | 0 |
| 8. | 8 | 0 | 0 | 0 |
| 9. | Unknown | 3 | 3 | 2 |

**65. Number of Sisters Schizophrenic (deteriorating illness)**

| | | | | |
|---|---|---|---|---|
| 0. | None | 194 | 118 | 201 |
| 1. | 1 | 4 | 0 | 1 |
| 2. | 2 | 0 | 0 | 0 |
| 3. | 3 | 0 | 0 | 0 |
| 4. | 4 | 0 | 0 | 0 |

| | | | | |
|---|---|---|---|---|
| 5. | 5 | 0 | 0 | 0 |
| 6. | 6 | 0 | 0 | 0 |
| 7. | 7 | 0 | 0 | 0 |
| 8. | 8 | 0 | 0 | 0 |
| 9. | Unknown | 2 | 4 | 1 |

**66. Number of Brothers Alcoholic**

| | | | | |
|---|---|---|---|---|
| 0. | None | 192 | 111 | 190 |
| 1. | 1 | 7 | 5 | 11 |
| 2. | 2 | 0 | 2 | 0 |
| 3. | 3 | 0 | 1 | 0 |
| 4. | 4 | 0 | 0 | 0 |
| 5. | 5 | 0 | 0 | 0 |
| 6. | 6 | 0 | 0 | 0 |
| 7. | 7 | 0 | 0 | 0 |
| 8. | 8 | 0 | 0 | 0 |
| 9. | Unknown | 1 | 3 | 2 |

**67. Suicide in Siblings**

| | | | | |
|---|---|---|---|---|
| 0. | None | 198 | 117 | 186 |
| 1. | 1 Brother | 1 | 2 | 10 |
| 2. | 1 Sister | 0 | 0 | 4 |
| 3. | 1 Brother, 1 sister | 0 | 0 | 0 |
| 4. | 2 Brothers | 0 | 0 | 1 |
| 5. | 2 Sisters | 0 | 0 | 0 |
| 6. | 2 Brothers, 1 sister | 0 | 0 | 0 |
| 7. | 1 Brother, 2 sisters | 0 | 0 | 0 |
| 8. | 4 Or more siblings | 0 | 0 | 0 |
| 9. | Unknown | 1 | 3 | 2 |

**68. Number of Children**

| | | | | |
|---|---|---|---|---|
| 0. | None | 157 | 59 | 70 |
| 1. | 1 | 18 | 15 | 39 |
| 2. | 2 | 11 | 24 | 31 |
| 3. | 3 | 9 | 11 | 26 |
| 4. | 4 | 1 | 4 | 10 |
| 5. | 5 | 1 | 0 | 17 |
| 6. | 6 | 2 | 1 | 3 |
| 7. | 7 | 0 | 3 | 5 |
| 8. | 8 or more | 1 | 2 | 2 |
| 9. | Unknown | 0 | 3 | 0 |

**69. Psychiatric Illnesses in Children, Any Kind**

| | | | | |
|---|---|---|---|---|
| 0. | None | 192 | 114 | 183 |
| 1. | Affective disorder | 0 | 1 | 5 |
| 2. | Schizophrenia | 1 | 0 | 0 |
| 3. | Alcoholism | 0 | 0 | 3 |
| 4. | Affective disorder and schizophrenia | 0 | 0 | 0 |
| 5. | Affective disorder and alcoholism | 0 | 0 | 0 |
| 6. | Schizophrenia and alcoholism | 0 | 0 | 0 |
| 7. | Affective disorder, alcoholism, and schizophrenia | 0 | 0 | 0 |
| 8. | Other combinations or undiagnosed illness, personality disorder | 7 | 4 | 12 |
| 9. | Unknown | 0 | 3 | 0 |

**70. Illness on Paternal Side of Family**

| | | | | |
|---|---|---|---|---|
| 0. | None | 73 | 50 | 60 |
| 1. | Affective disorder | 12 | 7 | 18 |
| 2. | Schizophrenia | 6 | 2 | 1 |
| 3. | Alcoholism | 14 | 6 | 4 |
| 4. | Affective disorder and schizophrenia | 0 | 0 | 0 |
| 5. | Affective disorder and alcoholism | 2 | 1 | 1 |
| 6. | Schizophrenia and alcoholism | 1 | 0 | 0 |
| 7. | Affective disorder, alcoholism, and schizophrenia | 0 | 0 | 0 |
| 8. | Other combinations or undiagnosed illness, personality disorder | 27 | 8 | 10 |
| 9. | Unknown | 65 | 48 | 109 |

**71. Illness on Maternal Side of Family**

| | | | | |
|---|---|---|---|---|
| 0. | None | 79 | 54 | 59 |
| 1. | Affective disorder | 19 | 9 | 21 |
| 2. | Schizophrenia | 5 | 2 | 3 |
| 3. | Alcoholism | 11 | 1 | 3 |
| 4. | Affective disorder and schizophrenia | 0 | 0 | 1 |
| 5. | Affective disorder and alcoholism | 1 | 0 | 2 |
| 6. | Schizophrenia and alcoholism | 0 | 0 | 1 |
| 7. | Affective disorder, alcoholism, and schizophrenia | 1 | 0 | 0 |

| 8. | Other combinations or undiagnosed illness, personality disorder | 27 | 12 | 10 |
|---|---|---|---|---|
| 9. | Unknown | 57 | 44 | 103 |

| **72.** | **Education** | | | |
|---|---|---|---|---|
| 0. | No formal education | 2 | 0 | 0 |
| 1. | 6th Grade or less | 1 | 2 | 8 |
| 2. | 8th Grade or less | 36 | 24 | 67 |
| 3. | High school—did not graduate | 31 | 18 | 33 |
| 4. | 12th Grade | 56 | 33 | 49 |
| 5. | College—did not graduate | 50 | 22 | 31 |
| 6. | College graduate | 14 | 14 | 14 |
| 7. | Professional degree (M.S., Ph.D., M.D., etc.) | 8 | 6 | 0 |
| 8. | Trade school | 2 | 2 | 1 |
| 9. | Other | 0 | 1 | 0 |

| **73.** | **Precipitating Factors** | | | |
|---|---|---|---|---|
| 0. | None | 178 | 88 | 122 |
| 1. | Psychological | 8 | 10 | 37 |
| 2. | Physical | 6 | 13 | 10 |
| 3. | Social | 2 | 2 | 10 |
| 4. | Physical, psychological, and social | 0 | 0 | 2 |
| 5. | Postpartum | 5 | 7 | 7 |
| 6. | Menopause | 1 | 0 | 12 |
| 7. | Physical and psychological | 0 | 2 | 3 |

| **74.** | **Hospital Diagnosis** | | | |
|---|---|---|---|---|
| 0. | Manic-depressive, depressed | 0 | 16 | 115 |
| 1. | Manic-depressive, manic | 0 | 75 | 0 |
| 2. | Other manic-depressive | 0 | 13 | 11 |
| 3. | Involutional melancholia, involutional psychosis, other | 1 | 5 | 62 |
| 4. | Other diagnoses (undiagnosed, neurosis, neurasthenia, psychopathic personality, paranoid condition) | 10 | 11 | 15 |
| 5. | Simple schizophrenia dementia praecox (DP) | 14 | 1 | 0 |
| 6. | Paranoid schizophrenia (DP) | 55 | 0 | 0 |
| 7. | Hebephrenic schizophrenia (DP) | 70 | 0 | 0 |

| | | | | |
|---|---|---|---|---|
| 8. | Catatonic schizophrenia (DP) | 5 | 1 | 0 |
| 9. | Other unspecified schizophrenia (DP) | 45 | 0 | 0 |

**75. Length of Follow-Up (last date with solid information)**

| | | | | |
|---|---|---|---|---|
| 0. | None | 9 | 8 | 12 |
| 1. | 1 Month | 5 | 4 | 8 |
| 2. | 3 Months | 10 | 10 | 9 |
| 3. | 6 Months | 25 | 15 | 22 |
| 4. | 1 Year | 62 | 41 | 58 |
| 5. | 2 Years | 27 | 14 | 6 |
| 6. | 3 Years | 32 | 4 | 14 |
| 7. | 5 Years | 14 | 14 | 39 |
| 8. | 10 Years | 12 | 8 | 26 |
| 9. | 20 Years | 4 | 4 | 9 |

**76. Quality of Follow-Up Information**

| | | | | |
|---|---|---|---|---|
| 0. | No follow-up | 9 | 8 | 11 |
| 1. | Patient seen here | 3 | 8 | 7 |
| 2. | Patient seen here plus subsequent information | 6 | 5 | 10 |
| 3. | Personal interview with patient | 25 | 11 | 12 |
| 4. | Personal interview with relative or close friend of patient | 4 | 5 | 5 |
| 5. | Letter from other hospital | 91 | 42 | 64 |
| 6. | Letter from relative, friend, or patient | 46 | 30 | 64 |
| 7. | Letter from physician or social worker | 14 | 10 | 28 |
| 8. | Obituary or other news clipping | 0 | 2 | 1 |
| 9. | Other information | 2 | 1 | 1 |

**77. Last Known Location of Patient**

| | | | | |
|---|---|---|---|---|
| 0. | No information | 7 | 6 | 8 |
| 1. | Home | 69 | 84 | 134 |
| 2. | Hospital, noncontinuous | 49 | 16 | 25 |
| 3. | Hospital, continuous since index admission | 73 | 15 | 33 |
| 4. | Dead, natural causes | 0 | 1 | 1 |
| 5. | Suicide | 0 | 0 | 0 |

| | | | | |
|---|---|---|---|---|
| 6. | In military service | 1 | 0 | 0 |
| 7. | In jail, penitentiary, reform school | 0 | 0 | 0 |
| 8. | Other | 1 | 0 | 2 |

**78.   Name of Follow-Up Institution**

| | | | | |
|---|---|---|---|---|
| 0. | None | 27 | 28 | 73 |
| 1. | Independent | 43 | 16 | 37 |
| 2. | Mount Pleasant | 50 | 23 | 23 |
| 3. | Clarinda | 35 | 18 | 24 |
| 4. | Cherokee | 27 | 15 | 21 |
| 5. | Any combination of above | 2 | 3 | 1 |
| 6. | The Retreat | 1 | 7 | 5 |
| 7. | Other hospital in Iowa | 8 | 6 | 11 |
| 8. | Other hospital outside Iowa | 7 | 6 | 8 |

**79.   Outcome of Illness**

| | | | | |
|---|---|---|---|---|
| 0. | Unknown | 11 | 9 | 12 |
| 1. | Complete recovery, no recurrence (must have corroboration) | 8 | 27 | 71 |
| 2. | Complete recovery, at least one relapse, now well | 3 | 11 | 15 |
| 3. | Complete recovery, at least one relapse, ill at last report | 4 | 21 | 22 |
| 4. | Never well, but social recovery | 13 | 8 | 18 |
| 5. | Never well, socially unrecovered, but not deteriorated | 120 | 23 | 43 |
| 6. | Never well, deteriorated (must have a) inadequate verbal communication, b) lack of working capacity, and c) inability to care for self) | 23 | 1 | 4 |
| 7. | Unsure whether well, but social recovery | 12 | 13 | 12 |
| 8. | Unsure whether well, but outside hospital | 6 | 9 | 6 |

**80.   Type of Treatment in Follow-Up**

| | | | | |
|---|---|---|---|---|
| 0. | None stated | 174 | 106 | 168 |
| 1. | Barbiturates only | 0 | 0 | 2 |
| 2. | Other drugs (not 7 or 8) | 0 | 1 | 1 |
| 3. | ECT | 7 | 7 | 13 |

| | | | | |
|---|---|---|---|---|
| 4. | Insulin shock treatments | 6 | 0 | 2 |
| 5. | Metrazol | 9 | 6 | 12 |
| 6. | Other convulsive therapies or combination of convulsive therapies | 2 | 1 | 1 |
| 7. | Phenothiazines | 1 | 0 | 1 |
| 8. | Antidepressants | 0 | 0 | 2 |
| 9. | Other drug treatments or combinations | 1 | 1 | 1 |

**81. Last Known Diagnosis**

| | | | | |
|---|---|---|---|---|
| 0. | No further diagnosis reported | 91 | 62 | 127 |
| 1. | Manic-depressive, depressed | 0 | 9 | 38 |
| 2. | Manic-depressive, manic or mixed | 0 | 39 | 1 |
| 3. | Involutional melancholia, involutional psychosis | 0 | 1 | 27 |
| 4. | Other diagnoses | 4 | 3 | 5 |
| 5. | Simple schizophrenia | 3 | 0 | 1 |
| 6. | Paranoid schizophrenia | 38 | 2 | 1 |
| 7. | Hebephrenic schizophrenia | 23 | 2 | 0 |
| 8. | Catatonic schizophrenia | 23 | 4 | 3 |
| 9. | Other or unspecified schizophrenia | 18 | 0 | 0 |

**82. Patient Became Married Since Discharge**

| | | | | |
|---|---|---|---|---|
| 0. | No | 197 | 117 | 195 |
| 1. | Yes | 3 | 5 | 8 |

**83. Birth of Children or Additional Children Since Discharge**

| | | | | |
|---|---|---|---|---|
| 0. | No | 200 | 115 | 198 |
| 1. | Yes | 0 | 7 | 5 |

**84. Successfully Completed School Since Discharge**

| | | | | |
|---|---|---|---|---|
| 0. | No | 199 | 116 | 202 |
| 1. | Yes | 1 | 3 | 1 |
| 2. | Returned to school, still there | 0 | 3 | 0 |

**85. Military Service Since Discharge**

| | | | | |
|---|---|---|---|---|
| 0. | No | 197 | 122 | 202 |
| 1. | Yes | 3 | 0 | 1 |

**86. Job Type Since Discharge (include homemaker)**

| | | | | |
|---|---|---|---|---|
| 0. | No job since discharge | 143 | 58 | 71 |
| 1. | Higher job level than before admission | 1 | 2 | 10 |

| | | | | |
|---|---|---|---|---|
| 2. | Same job level | 29 | 46 | 91 |
| 3. | Lower job level | 13 | 3 | 5 |
| 4. | Unknown | 14 | 13 | 26 |

**87. Number of Subsequent Episodes Known**

| | | | | |
|---|---|---|---|---|
| 0. | None | 129 | 69 | 141 |
| 1. | 1 | 20 | 25 | 22 |
| 2. | 2 | 2 | 11 | 9 |
| 3. | 3 | 0 | 2 | 4 |
| 4. | 4 | 1 | 1 | 2 |
| 5. | 5 | 0 | 0 | 2 |
| 6. | More than 5 | 2 | 2 | 2 |
| 7. | Chronic | 42 | 11 | 15 |
| 8. | Unknown | 4 | 1 | 6 |

**88. Occupation of Proband (prior to index admission)**

| | | | | |
|---|---|---|---|---|
| 0. | Unemployed | 34 | 4 | 4 |
| 1. | Unskilled laborer | 35 | 8 | 18 |
| 2. | Semiskilled or skilled laborer | 12 | 7 | 12 |
| 3. | White collar or clerical | 28 | 13 | 15 |
| 4. | Small business or managerial | 1 | 5 | 8 |
| 5. | Professional | 29 | 22 | 9 |
| 6. | Homemaker | 31 | 39 | 98 |
| 7. | Student | 18 | 10 | 3 |
| 8. | Farmer | 11 | 14 | 36 |
| 9. | Unknown | 1 | 0 | 0 |

**89. Length of Index Hospitalization (from admission to parole or discharge, whichever is shorter)**

| | | | | |
|---|---|---|---|---|
| 0. | 0–7 Days | 3 | 2 | 4 |
| 1. | 8–14 Days | 11 | 4 | 10 |
| 2. | 15–21 Days | 40 | 16 | 20 |
| 3. | 22–28 Days | 34 | 17 | 36 |
| 4. | 29–42 Days | 37 | 37 | 62 |
| 5. | 43–56 Days | 22 | 15 | 32 |
| 6. | 57–90 Days | 34 | 24 | 28 |
| 7. | 91–180 Days | 17 | 7 | 10 |
| 8. | 181–270 Days | 2 | 0 | 1 |

| 90. | Patient's Condition at Discharge | | | |
|-----|----------------------------------|-----|-----|-----|
| 1. | Worse | 3 | 4 | 5 |
| 2. | No change | 164 | 62 | 87 |
| 3. | Mild improvement | 22 | 19 | 36 |
| 4. | Marked improvement | 8 | 31 | 61 |
| 5. | Well | 2 | 6 | 13 |
| 6. | Deceased | 1 | 0 | 1 |

| 91. | Father's Occupation | | | |
|-----|---------------------|-----|-----|-----|
| 0. | Unemployed | 5 | 1 | 2 |
| 1. | Unskilled laborer | 19 | 13 | 19 |
| 2. | Semiskilled or skilled laborer | 34 | 9 | 26 |
| 3. | White collar or clerical | 20 | 5 | 8 |
| 4. | Small business or managerial | 22 | 20 | 22 |
| 5. | Professional | 17 | 11 | 8 |
| 6. | Homemaker | 0 | 0 | 0 |
| 7. | Student | 0 | 0 | 0 |
| 8. | Farmer | 67 | 46 | 98 |
| 9. | Unknown | 16 | 16 | 20 |

| 92. | Treatment in Hospital | | | |
|-----|-----------------------|-----|-----|-----|
| 0. | None | 135 | 108 | 137 |
| 1. | Barbiturates only | 13 | 9 | 35 |
| 2. | Other drugs (hormones, vitamins, etc.) | 12 | 2 | 17 |
| 3. | ECT | 15 | 0 | 0 |
| 4. | IST | 25 | 2 | 0 |
| 5. | Metrazol | 0 | 1 | 12 |
| 6. | Other or combination shock | 0 | 0 | 2 |

| 93. | Number of Subsequent Hospitalizations (include if transfer) | | | |
|-----|-------------------------------------------------------------|-----|-----|-----|
| 0. | 0 | 30 | 26 | 69 |
| 1. | 1 | 134 | 65 | 105 |
| 2. | 2 | 20 | 22 | 17 |
| 3. | 3 | 9 | 5 | 6 |
| 4. | 4 | 5 | 2 | 3 |
| 5. | 5 | 1 | 1 | 2 |
| 6. | 6 | 0 | 0 | 0 |
| 7. | 7 | 1 | 1 | 0 |
| 8. | 8 | 0 | 0 | 1 |

| 94. | **Urban-Rural (at admission)** | | | |
|-----|-------------------------------|-----|-----|-----|
| 1. | Urban | 119 | 54 | 106 |
| 2. | Intermediate (small town) | 26 | 28 | 34 |
| 3. | Farm | 55 | 40 | 63 |
| 95. | **Deceased?** | | | |
| 0. | No | 193 | 115 | 186 |
| 1. | Dead, natural causes | 4 | 5 | 11 |
| 2. | Suicide | 3 | 2 | 6 |

# References

American Psychiatric Association: Diagnostic and Statistical Manual of Mental Disorders, 3rd Edition. Washington, DC, American Psychiatric Association, 1980

American Psychiatric Association: Diagnostic and Statistical Manual of Mental Disorders, 3rd Edition, Revised. Washington, DC, American Psychiatric Association, 1987

Angst J: Zur aetiologie und Nosologie endogener depressiver psychosen, eine genetische, Soziologische und Klinische Studies. Monogr ad Gesamtgeb d Neurol Psychiat Heft 112. Heidelberg, Springer, 1966

Angst J, Perris C: Nosology of endogenous depression, a comparison of the findings of two studies. Arch Psychiat Nervenkr 210:373, 1968

Baron M, Gruen R, Rainer J, et al: A family study of schizophrenic and normal control probands: implications for the spectrum concept of schizophrenia. Am J Psychiatry 142:447–455, 1985

Baron M, Risch N, Hamburger R, et al: Genetic linkage between X-chromosome markers and bipolar affective illness. Nature 326:289–292, 1987

Bertelsen A: A Danish twin study of manic depressive disorders, in Origin, Prevention, and Treatment of Affective Disorders. Edited by Schou M, Stromgren E. London, Academic Press, 1979, pp 227–239

Black D, Winokur G, Nasrallah H: Is death from natural causes still excessive in psychiatric patients: a follow-up of 1593 patients with major affective disorder. J Nerv Ment Dis 175:674–680, 1987a

Black D, Winokur G, Nasrallah H: Suicide in subtypes of major affective disorder. Arch Gen Psychiatry 44:878–880, 1987b

Bleuler M: The long-term course of the schizophrenic psychoses. Psychol Med 4:244–254, 1974

Bleuler M: The Schizophrenic Disorders. New Haven and London, Yale University Press, 1978, pp 1–529, pp 191–192

Böök J: A genetic and neuropsychiatric investigation of a north Swedish population with special regard to schizophrenia and mental deficiency. Acta Genetica (Basel) 4:1–100, 1953

Cadoret R, Woolson R, Winokur G: The relationship of age of onset in unipolar affective disorder to risk of alcoholism and depression in patients. J Psychiatr Res 13:137–142, 1977

Cassidy W, Flanagan N, Spelman B, et al: Clinical observations in manic depressive disease. JAMA 164:1535–1546, 1957

Chandler J, Winokur G: How antipsychotic are the antipsychotics? Ann Clin Psychiatry 1:215–220, 1989

Cheadle A, Freeman H, Korer J: Chronic schizophrenic patients in the community. Br J Psychiatry 132:221–227, 1978

Chiompi L: The natural history of schizophrenia in the long-term. Br J Psychiatry 136:413–420, 1980

Clancy J, Crowe R, Winokur G, et al: The Iowa 500: precipitating factors in schizophrenia and primary affective disorder. Compr Psychiatry 14:197–202, 1973

Clancy J, Tsuang M, Norton B, et al: The Iowa 500: A comprehensive study of mania, depression and schizophrenia. Journal of the Iowa Medical Society 64:394–396, 398, 1974

Coleridge ST: The rime of the ancient mariner, in Lyrical Ballads, with a Few Other Poems. Bristol, T. N. Longman, 1798

Coryell W, Tsuang M: Should non-Feighner schizophrenia be classified with affective disorder? J Aff Disord 1:3–8, 1979

Coryell W, Tsuang M: Primary unipolar depression and the prognostic significance of delusions. Arch Gen Psychiatry 39:1181–1184, 1982

Coryell W, Winokur G: Course and outcome, in Handbook of Affective Disorders, 2nd Edition. Edited by Paykel E. Edingurgh and London, Churchill Livingstone, 1992, pp 89–108

Coryell W, Zimmerman M: Progress in the classification of functional psychoses. Am J Psychiatry 144:1471–1473, 1987

Coryell W, Tsuang M, McDaniel J: Psychotic features in major depression: Is mood congruence important. J Affect Disord 4:227–236, 1982

Coryell W, Endicott J, Keller M: Rapid cycling affective disorder: demographics, diagnosis, family history and course. Arch Gen Psychiatry 49:126–131, 1992

Cox D: Regression models and life tables. Journal of the Royal Statistical Society B, 34:187, 1972

Crowe R, Clarkson C, Tsai M, et al: Delusional disorder: jealous and non-jealous types. Eur Arch Psychiatry Clin Neurosci 237:179–183, 1988

Davison K: Schizophrenic-like psychoses associated with organic cerebral disorders: a review. Psychiatric Development 1:1–34, 1983

Essen-Möller E: Individual traits and morbidity in a Swedish rural population. Acta Psychiatr Neurol Scand Suppl 100, 1956

Faris T, Dunham H: Mental Disorders in Urban Areas. University of Chicago Press, Chicago, 1939

Feighner J, Robins E, Guze S, et al: Diagnostic criteria for use in psychiatric research. Arch Gen Psychiatry 26:57–63, 1972

Goldstein J, Faraone S, Chen W, et al: Sex differences in the familial transmission of schizophrenia. Br J Psychiatry 156:819–826, 1990

Gottesman I, McGuffin P, Farmer A: Clinical genetics as clues to the "real" genetics of schizophrenia. Schizophr Bull 13:23–47, 1987

Guze S, Cloninger C, Martin R, et al: A follow-up and family study of schizophrenia. Arch Gen Psychiatry 40:1273–1276, 1983

Hagnell O: A Prospective Study of the Incidence of Mental Disorder. Lund, Sweden, Scandinavian University Books, 1966

Hagnell O, Tunving K: Prevalence and nature of alcoholism in a total population. Social Psychiatry 7:190–201, 1972

Harding C, Brooks G, Ashikaga T, et al: The Vermont longitudinal study, II: long-term outcome for DSM-III schizophrenia. Am J Psychiatry 144:727–735, 1987

Hollingshead A, Redlich F: Social Class and Mental Illness: A Community Study. New York, Wiley, 1958

Johnstone E, Owens D, Gold A, et al: Schizophrenic patients discharged from hospital: a follow-up study. Br J Psychiatry 145:586–590, 1984

Johnstone E, Owens D, Frith C, et al: Institutionalization and the outcome of functional psychoses. Br J Psychiatry 146:36–44, 1985

Johnstone E, Macmillan J, Frith C, et al: Further investigation of the predictors of outcome following first schizophrenia episodes. Br J Psychiatry 157:182–189, 1990

Kallman F: The Genetics of Schizophrenia. New York, JJ Augustin, 1938

Kathol R, Winokur G: "Organic" and "psychotic" symptoms in unipolar (UP) and bipolar (BP) depressions. Compr Psychiatry 18:251–253, 1977

Kendler K, Tsuang M: Outcome and familial psychopathology in schizophrenia. Arch Gen Psychiatry 45:338–346, 1988

Kendler K, Gruenberg A, Strauss J: An independant analysis of the Copenhagen sample of the Danish adoption study of schizophrenia, III: the relationship of paranoid psychosis (delusional disorder) and the schizophrenia spectrum disorders. Arch Gen Psychiatry 38:985–987, 1981

Kendler K, Gruenberg A, Tsuang M: Outcome of schizophrenia subtypes defined by four diagnostic systems. Arch Gen Psychiatry 41:149–154, 1984

Kendler K, Masterson C, Davis K: Psychiatric illness in first degree relatives of patients with paranoid psychosis, schizophrenia and medical illness. Br J Psychiatry 147:524–531, 1985a

Kendler K, Gruenberg A, Tsuang M: Psychiatric illness in first degree relatives of schizophrenics and surgical control patients. Arch Gen Psychiatry 42:770–779, 1985b

Kendler K, Gruenberg A, Tsuang M: A family study of the subtypes of schizophrenia. Am J Psychiatry 145:57–62, 1988

Kety S: Mental illness in the biologic and adoptive relatives of schizophrenic adoptees: findings relevant to genetic and environmental factors in etiology. Am J Psychiatry 140:720–727, 1983

Kety S, Rosenthal D, Wender P, et al: Mental illness in the biological and adoptive families of adopted individuals who have become schizophrenic: a preliminary report based on psychiatric interview, in Genetic Research in Psychiatry. Edited by Fieve R, Rosenthal D, Brill H. Baltimore, MD, Johns Hopkins, 1975, pp 147–165

Kushon D, Helz J, Lau K, et al: Delusions of parasitosis: an entomologist's view, in New Research Programs and Abstracts. Presented at the 144th Annual Meeting of the American Psychiatric Association, New Orleans, 1991, p 160

Langfeldt G: The prognosis in schizophrenia. Acta Psychiatr Neurol Scand Suppl 110:1–66, 1956

Leighton A: My Name is Legion: Vol I of the Sterling County Study. New York, Basic Books, 1959

Leighton D, Harding J, Macklin D, et al: The Character of Danger: Vol III of the Sterling County Study. New York, Basic Books, 1963

Lewis N: The constitutional factors in dementia praecox. Nervous and Mental Disease Monograph Series #35. New York, Nervous and Mental Disease Publishing, 1923, pp 1–133

Lindelius R: A study of schizophrenia: a clinical, prognostic and family investigation. Acta Psychiatr Scand Suppl 216:1–125, 1970

Lundquist G: Progress and course in manic depressive psychoses: a follow-up study of 319 first admissions. Acta Psychiatrica et Neurologica Suppl 35:1–96, 1945

McCreadie R: The Nithsdale schizophrenia survey, I: psychiatric and social handicaps. Br J Psychiatry 140:582–586, 1982

Medical Research Council: Report by the Clinical Committee: clinical trial of the treatment of depressive illness. Lancet 1:881–886, 1969

Mendlewicz J, Rainer J: Adoption study supporting genetic transmission in manic depressive illness. Nature 268:327–329, 1977

Milton J: Comus, in Poetical Works. London, J. M. Dent & Sons, 1909

Morgan R: Conversations with chronic schizophrenic patients. Br J Psychiatry 134:187–194, 1979

Morrison J, Clancy J, Crowe R, et al: The Iowa 500, I: diagnostic validity in mania, depression and schizophrenia. Arch Gen Psychiatry 27:457–461, 1972

Nurnberger J, Goldin L, Gershon E: Genetics of psychiatric disorders, in The Medical Basis of Psychiatry. Edited by Winokur G, Clayton P. Philadelphia, PA, WB Saunders, 1986, pp 486–521

Opjordsmoen S: Delusional disorder, I: comparative long-term outcome. Acta Psychiatr Scand 80:603–612, 1989

Perris C: A study of bipolar (manic depressive) and unipolar recurrent depressive psychoses. Acta Psychiatr Scand Suppl 194:15–44, 1966

Pfohl B, Winokur G: Schizophrenia: course and outcome in Schizophrenia as a Brain Disease. Edited by Henn F, Nasrallah H. New York, Oxford University Press, 1982a

Pfohl B, Winokur G: The evolution of symptoms in institutionalized hebephrenic/catatonic schizophrenics. Br J Psychiatry 141:567–572, 1982b

Pfohl B, Winokur G: The micropsychopathology of hebephrenic/catatonic schizophrenia. J Nerv Ment Dis 171:296–300, 1983

Pfohl B, Stangl D, Tsuang M: The association between early parental loss and diagnosis in the Iowa 500. Arch Gen Psychiatry 40:965–967, 1983

Price J: The genetics of depressive behavior, in Recent Developments in Affective Disorders. Edited by Coppen A, Walk A. Ashford, Kent, Headley Bros, 1968, pp 37–56

Purtell J, Robins E, Cohen M: Observations on the clinical aspects of hysteria: a quantitive study of 50 patients and 156 control subjects. JAMA 146:902–909, 1951

Quitkin F, Rifkin A, Tsuang M, et al: Can schizophrenia with premorbid asociality be genetically distinguished from the other forms of schizophrenia? Psychiatry Res 2:99–105, 1980

Reich T, Clayton P, Winokur G: Family history studies, V: the genetics of mania. Am J Psychiatry 125:1358–1360, 1969

Robins E, Murphy G, Wilkinson R, et al: Some clinical considerations in the prevention of suicide based on a study of 134 successful suicides. Am J Public Health 49:888–899, 1959

Robins L, Helzer J, Weissman M, et al: Lifetime prevalence of specific psychiatric disorders in three sites. Arch Gen Psychiatry 41:949–958, 1984

Rogers K, Winokur G: The genetics of schizoaffective disorder and the schizophrenia spectrum, in Handbook of Schizophrenia, Vol 3: Nosology, Epidemiology, and Genetics of Schizophrenia. Edited by Tsuang M, Simpson J. Amsterdam, Elsevier, 1988, pp 481–500

Saran B: Lithium. Lancet 1:1208–1209, 1969

Schulsinger F, Kety S, Rosenthal D, et al: A family study of suicide, in Origin, Prevention, and Treatment of Affective Disorders. Edited by Schou M, Stromgren E. London, Academic Press, 1979, pp 277–287

Schulz B: Zur erbpathologie der schizophrenia. Zeitschrift für die Gesamte Neurologie und Psychiatrie 143:175–293, 1932

Slater E, Cowie V: The Genetics of Mental Disorders. London, Oxford University Press, 1971

Spitzer RL, Endicott J, Robins E: Research Diagnostic Criteria: rationale, and reliability. Arch Gen Psychiatry 35:773–782, 1978

Srole L: Measurements and classification in socio-psychiatric epidemiology: Midtown Manhattan study I (1954) and Midtown Manhattan study II (1975). J Health Soc Behav 16:347–364, 1975

Stephens J, Astrup C, Mangrum J: Prognostic factors in recovered and deteriorated schizophrenics. Am J Psychiatry 122:1116–1120, 1960

Thompson W, Orvashal H, Prusoff B, et al: An evaluation of the family history method for obtaining psychiatric disorders. Arch Gen Psychiatry 39:53–58, 1982

Tolstoy L: Anna Karenin. New York, W. W. Norton, 1970

Tsuang M: Schizophrenia syndromes: the search for subgroups in schizophrenia with brain dysfunction, in Schizophrenia as a Brain Disease. Edited by Henn F, Nasrallah H. London, Oxford University Press, 1982, pp 14–25

Tsuang M: Risk of suicide in the relatives of schizophrenics, manics, depressives and controls. J Clin Psychiatry 44:396–400, 1983

Tsuang M, Dempsey GM: Long-term outcome of major psychoses, II: "schizoaffective" disorder compared with schizophrenia, affective disorders, and a surgical control group. Arch Gen Psychiatry 36:1302–1304, 1979

Tsuang M, Winokur G: Criteria for subtyping schizophrenia: clinical differentiation of hebephrenic and paranoid schizophrenia. Arch Gen Psychiatry 31:43–47, 1974

Tsuang M, Winokur G: The Iowa 500: preliminary results of field work in a 35 year follow-up of depression, mania and schizophrenia. Canadian Psych Assoc J 20:359–364, 1975

Tsuang M, Woolson R: Mortality in patients with schizophrenia, mania, depression and surgical conditions: a comparison with general population mortality. Br J Psychiatry 130:162–166, 1977

Tsuang M, Woolson R: Excess mortality in schizophrenic and affective disorders: do suicides and accidental deaths solely account for this excess? Arch Gen Psychiatry 35:1181–1185, 1978

Tsuang M, Dempsey M, Rauscher F: A study of "atypical schizophrenia." Arch Gen Psychiatry 33:1157–1160, 1976

Tsuang M, Crowe R, Winokur G, et al: Relatives of schizophrenics, manics, depressives, and controls: an interview study of 1331 first-degree relatives, in The Nature of Schizophrenia. Edited by Wynne LC, Cromwell RL, Matthysse S. New York, Wiley, 1978, pp 52–58

Tsuang M, Woolson R, Fleming J: Long-term outcome of major psychoses; I: Schizophrenia and affective disorders compared with psychiatrically symptom-free surgical conditions. Arch Gen Psychiatry 36:1295–1301, 1979

Tsuang M, Woolson R, Fleming J: Causes of death in schizophrenia and manic-depression. Br J Psychiatr 136:239–242, 1980a

Tsuang M, Winokur G, Crowe R: Morbidity risks of schizophrenia and affective disorders among first degree relatives of patients with schizophrenia, mania, depression and surgical conditions. Br J Psych 137:497–504, 1980b

Tsuang M, Woolson R, Simpson J: The Iowa Structured Psychiatric Interview: rationale, reliability and validity. Acta Psych Scand Suppl 62:1–58, 283, 1980c

Tsuang M, Woolson R, Fleming J: Premature death in schizophrenia and affective disorders: an analysis of survival curves and variables affecting the shortened survival. Arch Gen Psychiatr 37:979–983, 1980d

Tsuang M, Woolson R, Fleming J: Schizophrenia and cancer death. Lancet 1:480–481, 1980e

Tsuang M, Woolson R, Simpson J: An evaluation of Feighner criteria for schizophrenia and affective disorders using long-term outcome data. Psychol Med 11:281–287, 1981a

Tsuang M, Woolson R, Winokur G, et al: Stability of psychiatric diagnosis: schizophrenia and affective disorder followed-up over a 30–40 year period. Arch Gen Psychiatry 38:535–539, 1981b

Tsuang M, Bucher K, Fleming J: Testing the monogenic theory of schizophrenia: an application of segregation methods of analysis to blind family study data. Br J Psychiatry 140:595–599, 1982

Tsuang M, Bucher K, Fleming J: A search for "schizophrenia spectrum disorders": an application of the multiple threshold model to blind family study data. Br J Psychiatry 143:572–577, 1983a

Tsuang M, Perkins K, Simpson J: Physical diseases in schizophrenia and affective disorders. J Clin Psychiatry 44:42–46, 1983b

Tsuang M, Winokur G, Crowe R: Psychiatric disorders among relatives of surgical controls. J Clin Psychiatry 45:420–422, 1984

Valliant G: Prospective prediction of schizophrenic remission. Arch Gen Psychiatry 11:509–518, 1964

Wheeler E, White P, Reed E, et al: Neurocirculatory asthenia (anxiety, neurosis, effort syndrome, neuroasthenia). JAMA 142:878–888, 1950

Wing JK, Cooper JE, Sartorius N: The Description and Classification of Psychiatric Symptoms: An Instruction Manual for the PSE and Catego System. London, Cambridge University Press, 1974

Winokur G: The types of affective disorders. J Nerv Ment Dis 156:82–97, 1973a

Winokur G: The Iowa 500: follow up of 225 depressives. Br J Psychiatry 123:543–548, 1973b

Winokur G: Diagnostic stability over time in schizophrenia, mania and depression. N Engl J Med 290:1027, 1974a

Winokur G: Genetic and clinical factors associated with course in depression. Pharmakopsychiatrie Neuro-psychopharmakologie 7:122–126, 1974b

Winokur G: Relationship of genetic factors to course and drug response in schizophrenia, mania, and depression, in Genetics and Psychopharmacology: Modern Problems in Pharmacopsychiatry. Edited by Mendlewicz J. Basel, Karger, 1975a, pp 1–11

Winokur G: The Iowa 500: heterogeneity and course in manic depressive illness (bipolar). Compr Psychiatry 16:125–129, 1975b

Winokur G: Delusional disorder (paranoia). Compr Psychiatry 18:511–521, 1977

Winokur G: Familial (genetic) subtypes of pure depressive disease. Am J Psychiatry 136:911–913, 1979

Winokur G: Controversies in depression or do clinicians know something after all? in Treatment of Depression: Old Controversies and New Approaches. Edited by Clayton P, Barrett J. New York, Raven, 1983, pp 153–167

Winokur G: Psychosis in bipolar and unipolar affective illness with special reference to schizoaffective disorder. Br J Psychiatry 145:236–242, 1984

Winokur G: Familial psychopathology in delusional disorder. Compr Psychiatry 26:241–248, 1985

Winokur G: Classification of chronic psychoses including delusional disorders and schizophrenia. Psychopathology 19:30–34, 1986

Winokur G: The schizoaffective continuum: Euclid's second axiom. Ann Clin Psychiatry 1:19–24, 1989

Winokur G: Mania and Depression: A Classification of Syndrome and Disease. Baltimore, MD, Johns Hopkins University Press, 1991

Winokur G, Clayton P: Family history studies, I: two types of affective disorders separated according to genetic and clinical factors, in Recent Advances in Biological Psychiatry, Vol IX. The Proceedings of the 21st Annual Convention and Scientific Program of the Society of Biological Psychiatry, Washington, DC, June 10–12, 1966. Edited by Wortis J, New York, Plenum, 1967, pp 35–50

Winokur G, Coryell W: Familial alcoholism in primary unipolar depressive disorder. Am J Psychiatry 148:184–188, 1991

Winokur G, Crowe R: Bipolar illness, the sex-polarity effect in affectively ill family members. Arch Gen Psychiatry 40:57–58, 1983

Winokur G, Morrison J: The Iowa 500: follow-up of 225 depressives. Br J Psychiatry 123:543–548, 1973

Winokur G, Tsuang M: A clinical and family history comparison of good outcome and poor outcome schizophrenia. Neuropsychobiology 1:59–64, 1975a

Winokur G, Tsuang M: Elation versus irritability in mania. Compr Psychiatry 16:435- 436, 1975b

Winokur G, Tsuang M: The Iowa 500: suicide in mania, depression and schizophrenia. Am J Psychiatry 132:650–651, 1975c

Winokur G, Tsuang M: Expectancy of alcoholism in a midwestern population. J Stud Alcohol 39:1964–1967, 1978

Winokur G, Tsuang M: Paranoid Versus Non-Paranoid Schizophrenia: definition and association, in Biological Psychiatry. Edited by Perris C, Struve G, Jansson B. Amsterdam, Elsevier, 1981, pp 761–765

Winokur G, Wesner R: From unipolar depression to bipolar illness: twenty-nine who changed. Acta Psychiatr Scand 76:59–63, 1987

Winokur G, Clayton P, Reich T: Manic Depressive Illness. St. Louis, MO, CV Mosby, 1969

Winokur G, Cadoret R, Dozab J, et al: Depressive disease, a genetic study. Arch Gen Psychiatry 24:135–144, 1971

Winokur G, Morrison J, Clancy J, et al: The Iowa 500, II: a blind family history comparison of mania, depression and schizophrenia. Arch Gen Psychiatry 27:462–464, 1972

Winokur G, Morrison J, Clancy J, et al: The Iowa 500: familial and clinical findings favor two kinds of depressive illness. Compr Psychiatry 14:99–106, 1973

Winokur G, Morrison J, Clancy J, et al: The Iowa 500: the clinical and genetic distinction of hebephrenia and paranoid schizophrenia. J Nerv Ment Dis 159:12–19, 1974

Winokur G, Tsuang M, Crowe R: The Iowa 500: affective disorder in relatives of manic and depressed patients. Am J Psychiatry 139:209–212, 1982

Winokur G, Dennert J, Angst J: Independent familial transmission of psychotic symptomatology in the affective disorders or does delusional depression breed true. Psychiatria Fennica 17:9–16, 1986

Winokur G, Pfohl B, Tsuang M: A 40-year follow-up of hebephrenic/catatonic schizophrenia in schizophrenia and aging, in Schizophrenia and Aging. Edited by Miller N, Cohen G., New York, Guilford, 1987, pp 52–60

Woolson RF, Tsuang MT, Urban LR: Data management in an epidemiological study: experiences from the Iowa 500 field follow-up and family study. Methods Inf Med 19:37–41, 1980

Wordsworth W: Lines, composed a few miles above Tintern Abbey, in Lyrical Ballads, With a Few Other Poems. Bristol, T. N. Longman, 1798

World Health Organization: The International Pilot Study of Schizophrenia. Geneva, Switzerland, World Health Organization, 1973, pp 67–77

World Health Organization: Mental Disorders: Glossary and Guide to Their Classification in Accordance With the Ninth Revision of the International Classification of Diseases. Geneva, Switzerland, World Health Organization, 1978

# Index

*Page numbers printed in **boldface** type refer to tables or figures.*